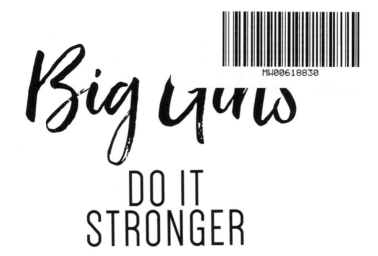

Big Girls

DO IT
STRONGER

The #wilderway 2.0:
move it and lose it!

Practical advice about all the most important
things in life, and my continuing journey
toward better health and happiness.

Jasinda Wilder

To Ru and Ree: Thank you for always pushing me to be the best example of a woman I can be for you. Mommy loves you.

I'm a married 42-year-old mother of four teenagers, and I have struggled with my weight for as long as I can remember. I have been following the Wilder Way since May 2016 and can truly say it has changed my life!! I am happier and healthier than I have ever been. I still have a ways to go with my weight, but I know that it will slowly come off. I am now able to run—yes, I said run—3 miles easily, and I actually *enjoy* running. My family is not completely on board, but they have definitely made some changes. I truly thank Coach J from the bottom from my now healthy heart. I feel like I finally have my life back!!

—Shari H

Six years ago I got news that woke me up. I had gone in for some tests, and the doctor informed me that some of them were border-line. A few days later he called and said the dreaded words: "If you lose some weight . . ." What came after that, though, was eye opening. He told me all about the things I could avoid if I'd just lose the weight, the pills I could stop taking, the machines I wouldn't need, the pain that would most likely go away. That phone call lit a fire under my butt, and I started the long process of losing weight. What I failed to realize was that dieting wasn't going to cut it. I could diet all I wanted, but it wasn't going to obtain the goals I had set for myself. I will say that I was mostly successful with my dieting. I lost about 40lbs in six years, and I kept all my weight off. I wasn't healthy, though.

May 2016 is when my life changed forever. I grabbed a copy of *Big*

Girls Do It Running, and I decided to give the program a try. I joined the Facebook group, and I thought I'd see what could happen. I was worried my husband wouldn't be on board, but he shocked me when he said he was all for the changes and to go ahead and make the changes we needed. Over the next eight weeks I found that I was sleeping better, I felt better, and the Coke I didn't think I could ever give up was just a distant thought.

Since I started the program, I've lost weight, a good bit, but I don't even care about the weight so much any more. I'm 37 years old, and I'm the healthiest I've been in my whole life. I was active in high school and as a kid, so that's saying something. I am active, and I eat well. This isn't a diet, it's a *lifestyle* I now live. I'm no longer thinking about things in terms of what I can't have, but I look at everything I can have, and I don't miss all the junk I used to think I couldn't live without. My husband has a saying: "Don't ask someone to do what you won't do yourself." I think of that every time I drag my feet when it's time to run. I am setting an example for my family, my kids, my parents, my sister, my friends. I want them to look at me and know that being healthy doesn't mean you have to diet your whole life. It doesn't mean you have to give up anything. You can live a full, active life and be happy and healthy doing it. I can't thank Jasinda enough for giving me my life back. When I look in the mirror I'm starting to like what I see. When my husband tells me I look good, I believe him now. This lifestyle isn't always easy, but it's the best thing that I've given to myself and to my family.

—Emily R

I'm 61 years old and I've gained and lost the same 30 or so pounds for decades. I'm really good at losing weight . . . I've had lots of practice. I've done shakes, extreme restriction, no carb, you name it, but I ALWAYS gained the weight back. Since reading BGDIR something has changed. I understand for the first time this is a daily life choice. Jasinda's recommendations make sense to me and her postings provide consistent support and ongoing motivation!

—Kim M

My girlfriend told me to read *Big Girls Do It Running* and join her 8-week challenge. I told her I don't run. She said I should just read the book. I'm not a big reader unless it's interesting, so I got the eBook and read it in about two weeks. Immediately I was very eager to give her challenge a try. I loved how it was a slow and steady process, not cold turkey. You slowly took out processed foods and sugars. That's what made it doable. I have lost 35 pounds so far!! I would not have been able to do that without Jasinda and the Wilder Way! It's been life changing. I am forever grateful to Jasinda for sharing her journey!! Much love!

—Richard C

Before adopting these changes, my health didn't matter to me. I wasn't concerned about getting bigger because I was already big. I wasn't taught how to manage my eating—or how vital exercise is. But I got a rude awakening when I went to my doctor's appointment. "You're on the verge of getting diabetes. You need to change your eating or something else . . . get into a program like Weight Watchers. I don't care. I want to see a change the next time I see you." A change . . . change was foreign to me, and I didn't want it. But I would try. So I did. Yet, it didn't last very long. So I did it again. But that time, I had my brother telling me I couldn't do it and I didn't want to do it anymore, so I stopped. I began over-eating again! And eating badly . . . I was never going to change, I'd think. The thing about change is if you're thinking negatively, you won't. If you give up before you start, you won't have a chance in the first place. I found the book through Jasinda's author page. I was amazed and inspired at her transformation. I then proceeded to purchase the book. Best money I ever spent! That was four months ago, and I'm down 30 lbs! I struggle some days like during my cycle or when I'm sick, because my cravings go haywire, but I know what I want. I know what it takes to get there. And I want to make that happen. Life is ten times better now than it was before. Thank you, Jasinda. You are an amazing person. I'm excited to see what the future holds!

—Dia L

Big Girls Do It Running helped me have the courage to say "I CAN DO THIS!" My first thought was, "How can this be any different from any of the other things I've tried?" Oh, but it *is* different. It has truly changed the way I look at food and how it affects my health. I have struggled with my weight since my son was born in 2001. I weighed 204 pounds when I started the 8-week challenge. I wouldn't say I had any health issues, but I was certainly headed that way. I now know a healthier way to live my life. It's all in the choices we make. I choose to be healthier. I really thought I would miss all the sugar-filled things. I simply don't! Stevia is my friend. My kids even call me Mrs. Stevia. Haha! I look forward to exercising. I actually love to get my wog on—#WoggingRocks! Through this journey I have also learned to LOVE ME. I am so proud of myself for all the work I've put in. I have lost 40 pounds and 9 inches off my waist since I began this journey to a healthier me. I now feel so energetic and alive.

—Christie aka Mrs. Stevia

Thanks so much, Jasinda, for all the work you put into BGDIR. Without you and the book I'd probably still be living an unhealthy lifestyle.

—Christie A

The Wilder Way has changed my life in too many ways to count. I have lost 50 pounds by following the Wilder Way. I have a ton of energy and my self-confidence is through the roof. My family is eating healthier foods and really enjoying them. My mom, dad, and several of my co-workers and friends are all eating The Wilder Way and are seeing huge results in weight loss and are just feeling better. The Wilder Way just makes sense and is very easy to follow, which is why it works. Thank you again for sharing your weight loss secret to success with all of us.

—Kelley J

Doing the Wilder Way program was not as difficult as I expected. It was manageable and realistic, and I never felt hungry! My body feels the changes, and I am so thankful that I feel healthier, look healthier, and lost some weight. It's a lifestyle that I'm happy I chose. Thank You, Jasinda!

—Marisol C

In May 2016, I grabbed *Big Girls Do It Running* and began reading the book that would change my life! I had met with my doctor about getting bypass surgery as my weight had hit 276, and I'm only 5'2" . . . he denied me because he doesn't believe in that procedure, and I felt hopeless! Along came Jasinda Wilder's book, and I had seen pictures of her changes so I thought, "Why not?" I am now down to 201.8 lbs! But more importantly my son and I have *REVERSED* our Type 2 diabetes!! My depression and anxiety are pretty much nonexistent and my son's Intermittent explosive disorder is under such control that I'm able to actually have a relationship with him and enjoy spending time with him (we've only had 1 meltdown since he started The Wilder Way in late June). And I have suffered from Crohn's Disease for years that no meds have been able to help me control . . . and guess what? I'm not taking ANY meds and haven't had ANY issues since after the first month!! Back pains I suffered from are gone and my energy levels are through the roof! I have my LIFE BACK—as a 42-year-old I no longer feel like a 80-year-old needing to lie in bed on a heating pad and medicate herself. Instead, I'm out running 5Ks (yup, 5 of them so far!). I enjoy going to the gym and actually living and laughing and participating in my life! I owe it all to #WilderWay, the *Big Girls Do It Running* book, and to Jasinda Wilder herself for sharing her book! It changed the lives of both my son and me—we have our lives back!!

—Dawn R

I have been on a weight-related roller coaster all my life. One of the first memories about my weight was when I was in the 7th or 8th grade, and weighed 120 lbs, which was a lot more than my classmates. I consider myself an experienced dieter, knowing how to get the weight off when my state of mind says it's time. I seem to have lived my adult life on a three-year cycle and I can count having lost over 350 pounds during my multiple diet phases.

This latest time, starting January 2016, I set my mind to losing it once again. I had been quite successful before I started the Wilder Way, having lost 38 pounds. I was weighing and measuring, counting calories, walking 4-5 times a week.

I began to wonder what I could do to make it last. I'm really sick of gaining it all back. I am also three months away from turning 60, which makes me worry about my health, and the age related diseases that seem to run in my family—namely diabetes and Alzheimer's disease. A friend of mine joined the original 8-week group and told me how it had worked for her, and she loaned me her copy of *Big Girls Do It Running*, and it really struck a chord with me. I was excited to see how my health would change as I cleared the sugar out and eliminated the processed flours. I was a little nervous about saying no to sugar but have found it amazingly easy! Thankfully, my husband is supportive and embraced this change with me. I have lost an additional 22 pounds following the Wilder Way, which finally puts my BMI into a normal range, per the American Heart Association. I feel great about myself and can feel the spring in my step when I walk! My husband has also lost about 20 pounds because of our changes, bringing his cholesterol to near normal, and he feels healthier than ever, too. This really feels like a lifestyle that we can easily maintain. Thank you, Jasinda!

—Cindy M

Because of Jasinda and the Wilder Way, I found my happiness. I get up each morning feeling energized. I know the best choices to make. I am no longer comforted by food. When I am stressed, I go for a wog instead of to my couch. I catch myself smiling all the time. It has been the most rewarding lifestyle change. Day by day I discover something new about myself and I've become stronger and more confident. I've discovered so many things I CAN do that, in the past, I was terrified to try. I look forward to exercising, it's the best part of my day! I love seeing what my body can do and I have a drive to push my limits! I do push-ups, jumping jacks, and I dance!! No more tapping my foot as I sit on the couch! Thank you from the bottom of my heart!

—Donna K

There have been so many books out there and all seem to say the same things, but this one caught my attention, so I downloaded the eBook because I didn't want another diet book laying around. Actually, I loved what it said and decided to try it, so I ordered a print copy so I could mark in it and find things fast. I called my sister and said, "Let's do this, it makes so much sense!" So we started, and my husband joined me, too. Then in August I got my other sister on board. The Wilder Way is something we all love and it's working! It's all about being healthy and not trying to starve ourselves. Thanks so much for writing *Big Girls do it Running*!

—Carol K

Where do I start? I have struggled with my weight my entire life. I was a dancer but I never had the ballerina body. In 2012 I hurt my back and ended up in a wheelchair for three years. I gained a lot of weight and have been living a completely sedentary lifestyle. BGDIR got me up. It gave me confidence. I just recently learned how to walk again. I walk with a brace and always a short distance, and I never thought I could do any more than that. BGDIR brought me in contact with other girls like me. I ended up walking a few times I week. I ended up walking a 5K!!! I never in my wildest dreams imagined I could do that! I was also dancing (Fitness Marshall on YouTube) again!! Thank you for everything, Jasinda!! If I can do it with all of my health problems—I have asthma, autoimmune, and thyroid problems too—then anyone can!!

—Krystin S

Forward

Dear Reader,

I hope you had a chance to read the testimonials at the beginning of this book. It is stories like these that have encouraged me to expand my journey in health and wellness. Every day I am inspired by people who have taken The Wilder Challenge, and who have been able to improve their lives, and the lives of their families and friends.

These success stories have kept me going, and now I'm so proud to share my new book—*BIG GIRLS DO IT STRONGER*—with you.

You know I'm not a doctor; I don't even play one on TV. I'm just a normal woman, a mom like you who has been so confused by all the contradictory health information out there. I've made it my mission to research this topic in depth, not only to help my family and friends but, hopefully, yours as well.

We've all been failing at health for too long; I've been counting calories and watching my portions all of my life. Guess what? Last year I found an easier way—*Big Girls Do It Running*—and it actually works! It helped me break the chains of my often-destructive relationship with food.

My new book, *Big Girls Do It Stronger*, is part of my path to becoming *stronger*: physically, mentally, and spiritually. I want to be strong and healthy in ways I never have before. I've stumbled through life in pain from my struggles with food, and I deeply hope that sharing my story will help you discover news ways to be healthy, and new ways to be strong.

When I started on this journey two years ago, I never would have imagined where I'd end up. At that time, I was newly pregnant and just trying to figure out how I could improve the way I felt during my pregnancy and make sure I had a healthy baby. That health crisis, and the places it has taken me, and the subjects of study it has prompted, may be the most important work of my life. The stories of those touched by *BIG GIRLS DO IT RUNNING* have been absolutely amazing—the photos, the faces, the stories are beautiful impressions left upon me that I thank God for every single day.

Thank you for continuing to take this journey with me. Thank you for continuing to push and inspire me . . . thank you for continuing to push yourself. I can't wait to see where this takes us.

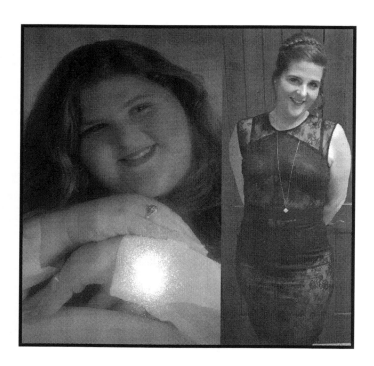

Author Note

Remember, *Big Girls Do It Stronger* is written from my personal perspective only, and the information contained herein should by no means be considered a substitute for the advice of a qualified medical professional.

Always consult your physician before beginning any new exercise or health program. Every effort has been made to ensure the accuracy of the information contained in this book as of the date of publication. The author and publisher (that's me!) expressly disclaim responsibility for any adverse effects arising from the use, or application, of the information contained herein.

Get Your Strong On!
Jasinda Wilder
March 2017

Contents

Chapter 1

FINDING MY STRONG:

The Swan Song of the Fat Girl

"It's not the destination, it's the journey."
—Missy Franklin

I'VE ALWAYS BEEN A TRENDSETTER. MY MOM SAYS I WAS A PUNKY Brewster type before anyone even knew who Punky was. I've always marched to the beat of my own drum. For example, if every other kid was screaming for chocolate ice cream, I would inevitably want blue moon—even if chocolate might have actually sounded better at the time.

I think most of it had to do with being a morbidly obese child. When you have that sort of problem, you either have to fit in or try to stand out in a way that makes it seem like you're confident, different, and bold. I used to think that maybe people would think I had made the choice to be fat on purpose; yeah, that was me, fat by choice, a trendsetter. At 12 years old I weighed nearly 300 pounds and stood almost six feet tall, so I already stood out like Mike Tyson in a neon pink scuba suit at a librarian convention. At that point why not twirl a baton while tap dancing and whistling Dixie? Everyone was already looking at me, right? At least that's how it felt inside my preteen body. I was often the biggest person in the room, so I might as well put bells on, too. I was going to be big and different, unique, a direct contradiction to the life I was handed. I was going to figure out some way to make being fat look cool. If my looks weren't going to get me in the door, I was going to make damn sure my shining personality and humor would. What flavor was my soul? Blue Moon.

I can't remember a time I ever felt strong; my legs always felt tired, my arms wouldn't support me . . . I was always just weak and slow. Slower than slow—I was part sloth. I remember in gym class— maybe 2nd or 3rd grade—we had to pull ourselves up a rope, a standard test in public school gym class. But for me it was a task the teacher knew she could not ask me to attempt. I was a manatee in gym class.

I never had enough rest, to the point that my body always just felt fatigued. Even at a time in my life when I was very active, I always felt like I was pushing my body to the point of near-collapse. Even just a few years ago, when I was traveling several times a month, I was frequently at the point of complete physical exhaustion.

Often, after doing a book signing or reader event, I would get invitations from readers and fellow authors to attend after-parties, and even though it always sounded fun, my body just wouldn't let me. My body was a mess, and I wasn't even thirty-five. So many nights after these events I would just cry while my husband consoled me, telling me it was okay and that readers would understand. But would they? Or would they just resign themselves to the fact that I was struggling physically? Did they know that I would much rather have a different body, one that would carry me to wherever all the fun was? How could *they* understand when even *I* couldn't? As my anger and pity consumed me, I would usually order room service, because the food would comfort me even when my husband's loving words couldn't. The cheesecake was always right.

There was one brief moment in my 20s when I did feel a tiny bit strong for about two seconds. I was a karaoke DJ at a bunch of local bars. I had a pretty decent show following, so people would come drink and dance and listen to me sing. This was right after I had my first big weight loss, so I was feeling pretty badass about myself. I'm not sure I was actually physically strong in any way shape or form—the emotional strength I was trying to portray was probably mostly just crap in a fancy package. I was still a mess—I was just a mess in a smaller size. There was one night in particular when I was feeling especially rough and tough, wearing a pretty tiny dress and black butt kicker boots. One of the men attending my show decided he was going to rough up his girlfriend in front of me and the rest of the bar patrons. I sat there for about two minutes before I jumped down from my booth, grabbed a pool stick from the wall, and stomped toward the gentleman, ready to beat him away from his girlfriend. Apparently the illusion of my strength was convincing enough that he let her go and he walked out.

That superhero moment felt pretty good—heck, it felt strong, it felt *amazing*. But deep down I knew even then that it was just the *illusion* of strength; what would real, authentic strength feel like? How would it look? How could that happen? Somehow I knew I had to wait a bit longer until I'd get my first real taste of it, but I knew it was coming—it was really just a question of when.

Now, there's a very real difference between physical and emotional strength, right? Let's just be honest about that. These things are both important but they are, at the core, dynamically different things. There have been plenty of times when I've felt emotional strength, such as when I gave birth to my children, or when I packed up my bags and left my abusive ex-husband; these were things that required emotional strength, but not necessarily physical strength.

In retrospect, it was almost as if my emotional strength was pushed to the limits throughout my life, but physically I wasn't really ever challenged. In fact, I didn't even think of myself as possessing any physical strength. At times in my life I questioned if I might be able to do something physical, only to give up easily. I remember trying to go for a run once and making it around the block before realizing it was a stupid idea—there's just no reason for a fat girl to run. Running is for humans who sport, and I *don't* sport.

My parents weren't real physically active people. I never thought of my father as weak, but he wasn't lifting weights or running. He moved if it was required for work, but he didn't pursue strength as a lifestyle; it just wasn't part of our lives.

Even when I was dancing, I didn't feel like I was ever really pushing my body or demanding more from myself. The teachers would look at me like I had some sort of disability and, really, I did, because even though I was a pretty accomplished dancer—I won several competitions—I just wasn't ever pushing my body. I would dance for a bit and then take a break, watch and learn and repeat steps, then take a break again. I never felt like an athlete when I was dancing. I didn't feel strong—mostly I just felt like a participant. It was fun, but it was a rare occurrence if I ever broke a sweat. And I do mean *ever*. Part of me wishes I could go back and try that all over again. What might have I achieved if I had pushed myself beyond those limitations?

What if someone had seen an athlete in me?

What if I had seen an athlete in myself?

When I got pregnant with my second daughter, body strength was honestly the furthest thing from my mind. I was a mother of five other children, a wife, a daughter, a *New York Times* bestselling author, and we were traveling all over the world signing books. Needless to say, it was a pretty busy life. I think at that point I had totally resigned myself to always having a body that would be the opposite of strong. I know some people might argue that it took physical strength for me to birth my children, but I guess in my mind that's something most human females can do . . . our bodies are naturally built to do it.

The kind of strength I was looking for was something different, something that, at the time, felt very unnatural to me. I wasn't even sure what it was or how I would get there, I just knew I wanted to be there so badly that nothing else really mattered. It was all connected to my health journey, and to my precious daughter. I needed to be strong not only for me, but for her, too. God was whispering in my ear to find it, to seek physical strength. Learn what my body can do, what it was created to do: run, push, pull, jump, and stretch.

And, finally, I think I was ready.

I needed to be mentally and emotionally ready to make the changes required to start my journey. When I was pregnant with my youngest daughter, something just clicked for me. I was sick of feeing sick—I wanted more from my body, I wanted to be as healthy and as strong as I could possibly be. At that point I didn't even know *what* was possible, but I just knew that I had to try for more.

I also think it takes a lot of strength to stay the course, to consistently want to make those healthy choices day after day. It isn't always easy, and you have to let go of the shackles holding you back. But you also have to *want* to be healthier and stronger, and you know hanging out with those old unhealthy habits is liking hanging out with people who bring you down.

Looking back, I think so much of my health struggle was simply a story in my head, comforting because it was familiar. Since I can't even remember a time when I felt "normal" or healthy, the idea of healthy was scary for me.

It might have been scary for you to even purchase this book, because it means there's a chance you might have to admit who you are, and you might try and fail. You might think there's no way you could ever really be strong—maybe you don't even know what that means in terms of your body and your health.

Ladies, I understand. This was scary for me too. My only reassurance for you is that, although this journey might not ever get any easier, you WILL get stronger. Day by day your body will do things that will amaze you. You will learn to love and appreciate it because, just like when you crossed the finish line after running your first 5K, you will feel empowered. When you're able to do some of the strength exercises shown later in this book, you will continue to be surprised by what is inside of you, and by the strength you possess.

I know where we're headed, and it's going to be an amazing ride! This beautiful bird is going to soar; this lion is going to roar! We can do this, together. Let go of the "I can't" and start chanting with me: "I can, I can, I can . . . I will, I will, I will . . . I am, I am, I AM!"

This is our new song, ladies.

In my mind I see that young girl, dressed in all her mixed-pattern glory, smiling at me, full of spunk and fire. I bet you can feel your inner little girl rooting for you, too. Let's do this. Let's get our strong on, and let's bring our sons and daughters with us.

Get Your Strong On!

Chapter 2

IF YOUR HUSBAND SAYS HE WANTS YOU TO LIFT HIS BIG BELLS, IT MIGHT NOT BE ABOUT SEX BUT . . . IT MIGHT.

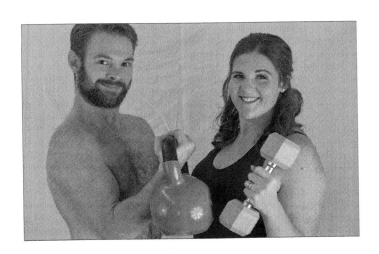

THERE WAS A DAY DURING THE FIRST WINTER OF MY HEALTH journey when my husband suggested I start lifting weights with him.

Now, let's take a step back and talk for a moment about Jack. Number one, he was always the nerdy little guy. When we met in college he weighed about as much as my left leg. He didn't have any muscles that I could see, and he certainly wasn't working out unless it had something to do with Dungeons & Dragons. I actually think our physical differences had a lot to do with why we didn't get together when we first met.

Neither of us could deny the close bond we felt the moment we met, but he was younger then, and so slim that I felt there was no way we could be a match. I know now just how stupid that was but, come on people, I was a dumb college kid and *My Giant Life* wasn't even a thing then.

Anyhoo, Jack didn't really start on his own physical journey until after I had started my quest for health and strength. Surprisingly, he didn't really fight me on it too hard, either. I remember during one of my back-to-back pregnancies our local church announced a charity 5K run, and I suggested Jack should try and run it. He actually laughed at me and told me he was, and I quote, "not an athlete." So we were both surprised when, number one, he actually did sign up to run it and number two, he didn't come in last. I don't even think he trained for it, he just went out and ran it, and did okay, surprising both of us, and him most of all, I think.

So when I told him I had decided I didn't want to live as I had my entire life, that I wanted something more, that I wanted a healthy and active life, he just agreed and told me he would be there with me for the ride.

When I started running I mostly did it by myself. I guess I needed that time to just focus on me and on the road without having to to worry about my husband or kids or work. I just wanted to have that peace, and the time to think without other distractions. Jack and I really weren't working out together except for when we did our big family runs. I had been doing some light kettlebell exercises that I had found on YouTube when I wasn't running, because I liked using the weights, and I always felt stronger after my kettlebell workouts—it was a different feeling than my running gave me.

Well . . . Jack asked me for his own set of bells for Christmas, because he wanted to start doing this Russian kettlebell training program he had found. He started training fast and hard, with crazy results. He was actually waking up at 5 AM to do these workouts, which shows just how much he loved them (insert eyeroll here). It was actually annoying for me to see how geeked out he was getting about his big, heavy bells.

But you'll hear more about Jack and his bells later. He's actually got a whole simple beginner kettlebell plan lined up for you later in this book! I'm sure you've guessed it by now, but Jack and I eventually started lifting the heavy bells together. I guess the couple who lifts kettlebells together stays together, right?

So, get ready friends. We want to get you tossing Jack's bells with us. Don't make any plans for the next few days—this is going to be good, I promise.

This book is going to incorporate what we talked about in BGDIR while taking your health and your strength to the next level. I want this book to work as a *BIG GIRLS DO IT RUNNING 2.0*: a way to add to, or revise, your original plan.

When I truly began feeling good I think it was a natural extension of my wellness to want to move. I LOVE (hate) to run, and I'll never stop unless Jack has to either drag me or wheel me over the finish line. I never plan to stop running, but I think there's also something to be said for strength training.

Jack and I don't belong to a gym, but we try to get a total body workout in our own home with just a few items. For less than you would pay for a year's gym membership, you can easily make a corner of your home just as effective as any gym. Even a very small space will work (just don't throw your kettlebells through an apartment wall).

If you have a friend, sister, husband, or child who is on this journey with you, this is something you can do with them, too. The plan Jack and I have come up with is something our 10- and 12-year-olds, their grandma, and Aunt Karri can all do, and it is even challenging for my Marine brother-in-law. In the same way anyone can run a 5k with you, anyone and everyone can join in for the fun of strength training exercises.

I also have some exciting new jump-start plans to build in some extra nutrition for strength training and, like the nutrition plans in BGDIR, they will be simple, fast, and nutritious.

Good nutrition provides at least 80% of your overall health, so we need to make sure that when you are doing these intense workouts with weights that you are getting proper nutrition, because your body will need MORE, not less. We need to feed our muscles.

I'm also going to tackle a few other important topics that have come out of the response to *BIG GIRLS DO IT RUNNING*. In this book I'm going to talk more about sex, food choice, portions, cheat days, skin, plastic surgery, active lifestyle, your kids and sex . . . and wine. All the most important things. Did I mention sex? Jack wanted to make sure that was fully covered—he'll have some input on that later, so stay tuned.

When I first wrote *BIG GIRLS DO IT RUNNING* I honestly had no idea how strong or positive the reader response would be. When the book was released in May of 2016 I was expecting to increase my social media presence, what with answering questions and leading the 8-week challenge, but I never thought I would be getting anywhere from five hundred to a thousand questions a day!

What this told me was: a) I had made the correct decision in putting myself out there with this book, and b) there was lots more information to add to further support of The Wilder Way plan. It has been so encouraging for Jack and me to have so many amazing interactions with our readers, to see how their lives have been changed so positively. I am so excited about what God is doing in my life, and one day I hope I can be an advocate for health and wellness on an even larger scale.

You're all part of my story, each and every one of you. We really hope and pray that this book will give you the additional tools you might need to further improve your life and health. No, we are not health experts or doctors or physical trainers, but we are two people who have researched, tried hard, and both failed and succeeded in this health and fitness maze.

Being busy, normal, stressed-out working parents, just like you, has given us some insight and experience as to what people want when it comes to the "quick and dirty" fitness plan most of us really need. We are excited about this next leg of the journey; let's get stronger together!

It's time to find our strong and embrace it and show our sons and daughters how amazing their bodies can be. If our daughters and sons can feel truly physically and emotionally strong, how much better would our world be?

You'll find that this book will give you a place to begin a new challenge regardless if you are a beginner, or if you've already been doing some strengthening and conditioning on your own, or if you're a pro. Jack and I really want to make sure that we can bring everyone along. We've even tested these exercises on our kids. If your children want to do these workouts with you, they absolutely can!

If you can't jump, no worries! You can modify this to make it work for you. If you're a walker, no problem! If you are working out with a trainer already, we have something here for you, too. Don't worry! Together, Jack and I will give you some new and old ways to work that new body.

Before we jump in and start lifting our weights, though, I want to share with you a few other stories, tips, and tricks that might also help you along your #WilderWay. Many of the chapters that follow came from the questions and observations from my *BIG GIRLS DO IT RUNNING* FACEBOOK GROUP. If you haven't joined that group yet, stop what you are doing right now and join. You'll find support from other members, answers to frequently asked questions, as well as videos from Jack and me that will help you along the way! There's everything in there from issues with sagging skin, to sprinting, to new recipes; we aren't leaving anything out.

There's so much we want to share with you, so grab a glass of Josh Cab Sav, put your feet up, and let's find our strong. It's about time!

Chapter 3

SKIN, SAGGING BOOBS, AND PLASTIC SURGERY: LIFTING UP MY GIRLS!

W E SHOULD JUST GET RIGHT INTO IT, SHOULDN'T WE? NOW, I'M warning you that some of this is a bit graphic and personal, so if hearing about my nipples makes you uncomfortable, just move on to the next chapter . . . or put a clamp on it.

When I had photographs taken for the cover of the first book, the photographer heard me complaining about the sagging skin issues I was having. She gave me the name of her plastic surgeon that, ironically, was the same person I'd heard about from someone local just a few weeks prior. At that point I really wasn't keen on the idea of having any plastic surgery done, as I had already had my fair share of surgeries, and I wasn't really interested in adding to the jigsaw puzzle of scars that was my body. My husband really didn't care either, and since I only ever got naked for him I figured it was better to just invest in good support garments. Everyone already knows how I feel about SPANX: they rock my world, and any woman with pounds-worth of hanging skin is going to agree with me on this.

Then, when I got the photos back from the photographer, I had a bit of a come to Jesus moment. Seeing myself in SPANX, on the cover made me feel like maybe I should at least meet with this surgeon and see what he had to say about the current state of my skin problems. I already knew running was causing major problems for my skin, even with using compression garments. So maybe it was worth talking about. I made the appointment and canceled it. Made it again and cancelled it again, and then finally made it one more time and actually showed up.

I've had some pretty scary and traumatic medical situations, so I was very, very nervous about my appointment with Dr. K; I even thought about having a glass of wine before my afternoon meeting, but, thankfully, Jack convinced me otherwise. Jack went with me, and I brought a list of things that were causing me discomfort or irritation as the welcome packet had suggested.

I was trying not to wog out of the office as I waited for him to come in, but I needn't have worried. Let me mention that if I was to create the perfect plastic surgeon for me, it would be Dr K—he has the most laid-back bedside manner ever, but he's a total perfectionist in the operating room. If you are going to have someone rearrange your body, you want someone who is so OCD that even his sock drawer is color coordinated. Right?

He took a very long look at my body, starting with my legs and ending with my boobs, which were at the very, very end of my list because I didn't think they were affecting my ability to run. After all the weight loss and gain, and loss and gain, and finally loss again, and then all the breast feeding, I had just resigned myself to the fact that my boobs would be DD windsocks hanging out near my knees unless I was wearing a very powerful and very expensive bra.

I'm not really sure why I didn't see another option, or why I wasn't that excited about a change in that region, but I guess because my legs were so chafed and painful they needed the most urgent attention. Maybe I had subconsciously given up on my boobs? They didn't really do much for me at this point. My legs, my arms . . . now *those* were doing something for me on a daily basis—and not always good. When I reflect back I feel a bit bad for my poor boobs; they weren't even really on my radar. But then when Dr. K looked at my list he suggested that I get totally naked so he could do his assessment—have I mentioned Dr. K isn't hard on the eyes?

So there I was totally naked with my husband and Dr. K in the consultation room—hey now, I know what you're thinking . . . get your mind out of the gutter, people! (insert eye-roll/giggle emoji here) Dr. K takes one look at my body and says "Nope, we need to do your boobs."

Boobs? *Really?* Did he have a secret meeting with my husband prior to his consult? Did he not see the total disaster that are my legs?

Over the next hour he reprioritized my list. He showed me pictures. He gave me the best possible scenarios and the worst. He listened to me. He said he would do whatever he could to make my body as functional as possible for what I wanted to do with it. Then he shook my hand and my husband's and walked out.

Which was when I took off my muted green hospital gown and started to cry. Now, I'm not at all a big crier—in fact, I'm one of those odd women who didn't even cry much during all of my pregnancies. But something about that meeting, something about talking about each part of my body and what it had been through had me in quite a state. I needed a glass of dry red wine, or two. Or three . . .

Jack, in his usual wonderful and lovely way, said that he would support whatever I wanted to do. He's the sort of husband who just wants me to be happy, probably at least in part because that usually means he gets more sex. He's pretty simple that way. So I told him

I wanted to think about it, pray about it, talk to my regular doctor about it, and also consult my good friend Google for horrible photos and videos . . . because that's what any normal person contemplating elective surgery does, right?

Now, I'm going to warn you that drinking wine while looking up said photos and videos IS NOT A GOOD IDEA! I ended up watching a video where some guy's nipples had to be taken completely off, and then they turned black and *DIED*. I'm not even joking. DO NOT look that up right now. Trust me, don't—it's horrible. I was sure the same thing would happen to me, that I'd be forced to live the remainder of my life without nipples, or with cadaver nipples, or pepperoni nipples . . . this was where my wine-soaked mind was wandering. So, I decided it might be a good idea to talk to my GP, Dr. P at my next appointment in a few weeks time. The Internet searches on this stuff were not helping.

Important side note: finding good doctors isn't always easy. It is time consuming for one thing, but it is ALWAYS worth it to make the extra effort. You want the best people giving you advice and suggestions about your body and health. *You* pay *them*, so don't settle for a doctor who wants to prescribe another pill. Find a doctor who is also concerned about your nutrition, your physical movement and strength. My primary care doctor, Dr. P, is the sweetest little thing. She's younger than I am and she did some of her medical school coursework in eating disorders and body image. She's wonderful, and absolutely what I need in a primary care physician.

Anyway, when I talked to Dr. P about my list and Dr. K's suggestions she completely agreed with him. I couldn't believe it. She said she believes that breast reduction and reconstruction is almost always a good idea if you are over a D-cup and/or have experienced significant weight loss. She said that of all the plastic surgery she's seen done, that a breast reduction has one of the greatest results. She also commented about how wonderful it would be for my running and my back.

I didn't really believe her, to be totally honest. My focus was always on my legs and lungs when I was running—my boobs never even entered the equation. I guess I just needed to think about it more. Did I really want to give up my amazing collection of super-strength bras? I already had all the matching panties. Would it really matter to me in the long run? Did I really have back issues I was ignoring? Or would they eventually appear? I just wasn't convinced. Why hadn't Dr. K just agreed with my leg plan? Why was everyone so keen on rearranging the windsocks? I was baffled.

So I waited until I was convinced. I would like to say I waited a week, but it didn't even take me that long. Jack and I were having marital time and both he and I were trying to maneuver the windsocks, which were sore from being chafed from running even while wearing one of the best running bras you can buy. This led me to the realization that this problem might be a bit worse than I had acknowledged. Ugh! So I called Dr. K to see if he would talk to me again.

I wanted to ask him about this black nipple/pepperoni thing face-to-face to make sure he hadn't ever done anything like that. Dr. K was shocked to hear about the black nipple video and I had to admit to him that I had been searching for these things on the Internet. When I told him it was from a reality TV show his face displayed some disappointment in me.

"Don't you watch reality TV, Dr. K?" I asked.

"No, I don't," he replied.

"Wow, Dr. K, you're missing out!" I said. "*THE REAL HOUSEWIVES* is a must watch."

He just smiled and nodded at me. I guess it might be a good thing that he doesn't have time for such things . . . he's busy golfing and restoring antique boats, you know, all the things normal plastic surgeons do, right? After he assured me that my nipples probably wouldn't die, I decided I wanted to go through with the breast reduction surgery. He also told me this procedure was by far the easiest. He said I wouldn't need much recovery time and figured it would only slow me down for a few days. Sounded good to me. Let's just ease into this, right?

The surgery took place in the early morning a few months later. Dr. K wasn't feeling great, but he was a trooper. He spent a good half hour on his knees in the prep room drawing all over my boobs until he had the perfect map to make things right. Now I bet some of you might be wondering at this point why in the world I'm sharing this story; it's so personal and so uncomfortable. Well, here's why.

This surgery, this act of bravery, gave me something I could have never imagined. Magic happened during that surgery. I came out a whole new woman. I know it sounds crazy, but having that surgery gave me so much that I felt the need to share, so other women who might consider this surgery for themselves will have a story from a friend that might give them comfort or support before making their decision.

Even when I walked in and lay down on the table, I didn't think this surgery was going to do much. Sure it might take some weight off, it might help with my under-boob irritation, and it might save me from back issues down the road, but I had no clue what having 44DD breasts for most of my life had really done to me, how they had literally weighed me down.

Of all of the surgeries I've ever had this was, by far, the easiest for me. So easy that I actually left the outpatient surgery center only an hour or two after it was complete. The pain was pretty minimal and I used some pain management, but not as much as I had expected. I spent the afternoon in my own bed resting, and by the next morning I was feeling pretty good. Now, I have to say that I think my pain tolerance might be a bit higher than most people's but, still, this wasn't bad AT ALL.

When the bandages finally came off and I looked up at my husband's big eyes and saw his two thumbs up, I could see that he was excited about it, too.

I couldn't run for several weeks because I was healing, so when I was finally able to get out and run I couldn't believe the difference in how my body felt. I didn't have the upper back pain I usually felt right when I would start out. My whole upper body felt so much lighter. I think I might have actually leapt a few times like a gazelle! During my first three-mile run with my new boobs I cut about three whole minutes off my average run time. I know that might not sound like a big difference, but to me it was HUGE. That and the way my body felt after running with the new girls caused me to break out into tears of joy.

The weight I lost from this surgery honestly wasn't much at all. Maybe a few ounces? But what I gained from that procedure was crazy. I felt like a totally new me, a lighter me. It might sound corny, but it wasn't just that I didn't have that heaviness on my chest, but I also lost a heaviness in my heart.

Those old boobs had been important to me even when they became very disfigured. Those boobs had fed my children, had been part of the body that loved my husband, they'd been with me in the highs and lows, they'd hugged friends and family, and they'd kept my hands warm at night, but these new boobs, these ones . . . they were fucking *aerodynamic*. These babies were Jasinda Boobs 2.0, and I was going to do things with them I couldn't even have imagined before. They were the start of finding my strong.

Thank you Dr. K, you were so right. Boobs for the win!

PRO TIP: If you decide you want to get some sort of surgical help, be sure to talk to several surgeons to see what they suggest, and ask lots of questions. This is really an art form, and each surgeon has slightly different ideas and approaches on what is best. I know I was surprised by some of the different advice I received.

Chapter 4

WHO IS THIS LADY, AND WHERE DID JASINDA GO?

"My grandmother started walking five miles a day when she was sixty. She's ninety-seven now, and we don't know where the heck she is."
—Ellen DeGeneres

WHEN I RELEASED *BIG GIRLS DO IT RUNNING* I GOT A BIT of flack for the title and the picture of me on the cover. Why? Well, I guess no one wants to run. Ha! Can you imagine that? But most of the negative feedback I got about the cover was that I still looked fat. Can you believe that?

Here's the deal: was I at my end point with my weight loss? NOPE! But I was at a place where I had steadily lost weight and was in a very healthy place? YES! And not just me, my whole family was getting healthy. So I was telling my story from that point. I was in that moment.

I guess in my head I was thinking that if people saw someone they could relate to on the cover, then they might pick it up. My agent even suggested changing the title and cover once it was released, but you can probably guess my answer to that: NOPE! If I'm going to put *my* name on the title of *my* book and publish it myself then I am going to put my silly butt in Spanx and show people that healthy doesn't have to look the way we think it does.

So, hey you, the person out there criticizing me and my body—when you can run a 5K in the dead of winter dragging a toddler with one hand while pushing a jogging stroller with the other, then we can sit down and talk about what you would rather have on the cover of my book (insert eye roll here).

The great thing about getting older, and having so many kids, and living the life I've had is that it takes a lot to ruffle my feathers. One of the only things that will piss me off is when someone tells me I can't do something. Trust me; don't even *think* about trying that with a mother of six—it won't go well for you.

As you can see, this book cover is similar to the cover for BGDIR: my healthy butt on the cover. Don't even try to convince me it isn't a great idea. I'm still working to change the way we think about how we look at health—more on that later, though . . . I'm getting ahead of myself.

As I'm writing this right now, BGDIR was only released six months or so, and so much has happened since then. At the release of *BIG GIRLS DO IT RUNNING*, my older kids, my husband and I all ran a 10K together. Wow, that was fun. I was so proud of my family, especially my three older kids who were only 10, 11, and 12 at the time. They all finished ahead of me, and they were there cheering me on as I ran into the stadium and across the finish line.

I will probably remember that day for the rest of my life. I didn't know we would be running into a stadium where people would be waiting to cheer on the finishers. They had a DJ with music blasting, and as soon as I wogged into the stadium they started playing

"MIAMI" by Will Smith.

I don't even know what came over me. I know every single word of that song! I LOVE THAT SONG! It came out the year I graduated high school, and it's my JAM! Come on, you remember how hot that track was, right? If you haven't heard it in awhile you should totally YouTube or Spotify it right now! It's still good!

I was so overwhelmed with happiness at that moment that I danced my butt to the finish line. I don't even know what the people in the stadium thought about me at that point but, in my mind, they were cheering me on. It felt like the stands were filled with all of my readers chanting "BIG GIRLS! BIG GIRLS!" and dancing with me to the finish. Yes, maybe I did need more oxygen and some electrolytes and, yes, it was entirely possible I was close to losing my mind. But, I actually didn't lose my mind. I got my *much*-smaller-than-it-was-in-1997 butt across the finish line and I cried. I couldn't believe I'd done it! I couldn't believe Will Smith was there singing "MIAMI" just for me. Okay, so he wasn't *really* there, but it did feel pretty cool to have that jam playing as I crossed the finish line.

I really hope you've experienced something like that on your own journey on the #WilderWay. I hope you've felt the joy of reaching your own finish line, that you now know it isn't about what your body *can't* do, it's about what it *won't* do if you don't even ask it to try.

I think of that moment so often. What if I had never asked my body to try this? Where would I be? Probably still sick, napping each day, in a sugar daze. But now? This amazing, powerful body of mine has run over a *dozen* 5K races, one *very* difficult uphill trail run, and a 10K. How awesome is that? Even just two years ago I would probably be getting ready for a nap right about now just to make it to 10 PM.

Yes, my life was busy then too, but the differences between then and now are really quite remarkable. And it didn't take special medication or a great spiritual quest. It took the simple realization that I wanted more from my life and more from myself and, let me tell you, nothing tastes better than the hope that life can be more.

Here's the awesome thing about hope: I think it multiplies, and it can be contagious.

The more my family keeps running, challenging ourselves, pushing ourselves, the more we all want. We want more of the good things we're feeling. Now, does that mean that every single day we wake up and lace on our running shoes? No way! But it has completely shifted our family life and the time we spend together. It's weird to me now that so many people think of our family as an "active family." We still don't watch much TV, we walk together, we hike, we swim, we run, we work out. It's not perfect, and it's usually messy, but it is something that I'm pretty proud of. Yes, we occasionally have to pull one of the toddlers some of the way, but when we get to that finish line, everyone is excited and feeling good.

When I first wrote *BIG GIRLS DO IT RUNNING* I had a tiny hope that other families would catch that same fire, and I got my wish. It was so neat to see so many other families sending me photos of them doing their 5K races together, all those big smiles on their sweaty, red faces. It was awesome! And I hope those same families will keep it up. Hey, maybe you can only do one race a year, but make it a healthy tradition that sticks. Maybe it's something you do on Thanksgiving, all dressed like a flock of turkeys. Maybe you take your daughter to a princess run sporting your tutu. Whatever it is, don't forget how good that first one felt. Don't let go of the bond your family makes when they challenge, motivate, and inspire each other toward better health. This is good stuff!

I think that finding your strong isn't always just physical—it's spiritual, it's mental, and it's deep down at the core of who we are. I think so many of us think we are weak. In fact, when I asked the *BIG GIRLS DO IT RUNNING* Facebook group when they had last felt strong, most of them said they *never* had. A few mentioned that when they gave birth they felt it for a few hours, or a day, or a week. Still, it was clear most of them were still waiting to find their strong.

Maybe we all just need a reason? Maybe we all just need that push, someone to tell us that we *can*; I know I need that every single day. I need someone to show up next to my bed each morning and whisper in my ear that yes, I *can* push, pull, lift, and run myself strong today (Please don't actually break into my house and do that, though).

When I was a teacher I was often surprised when a student told me they couldn't do something. Usually, I would have to tell them they could a few times and then bingo, they would do it. There's really something to be said for positive self-talk as well as reassurance from others. Once someone else tells you that you can achieve something, you usually can. If your mind sees you in that picture in your mind, if you envision yourself actually doing it, then a little seed of hope takes root and begins to grow. If you tell yourself you *can* deadlift that 150 lb barbell every single day, then guess what? There's a better chance of you eventually being able to lift it than if you're always telling yourself there's no way you could ever do it.

My whole life I hid behind negative self-talk. It would keep me from doing so many great things, exciting things, things that I might never get a chance to try again. I've been on four trips to amusement parks when I literally just sat and watched everyone else have fun. Not only could I not fit on most of the rides, but that fact alone hurt so bad I would be a depressed pony the entire time I was there.

I remember one time very vividly—it was my honeymoon from

my first marriage. My new husband loved rollercoasters and his grandparents had a condo near Orlando, so we drove down for a few days of fun and sun together. Although I should have been very happy, if you've read *BIG GIRLS DO IT RUNNING* you know that it was not one of the highlights of my life. I ended up being upset, full of regret, or crying almost the entire time we were in Florida. When we went to Hollywood Studios I just followed my new husband around and sat aside as he went on rides I couldn't fit on.

Even though we both knew by the second ride that I wouldn't fit on any of them, he still made me try. I'm not sure I can adequately express the amount of humiliation I felt in not being able to fit into the seats; and then, to make my mortification complete, at one point I got stuck and it took him and another man to get me out of the chair. I left one of the happiest places on earth feeling nothing like happy. I felt, at that point, at nineteen, that maybe I didn't even deserve happiness.

I have some wisdom I'd like to share today—at thirty-seven—to that nineteen-year-old girl: we all deserve happiness, dear. It's a choice—so choose it.

This past summer Jack and I traveled down to Florida with Nanny Karri (yes, *that* Nanny Karri), and my brother-in-law, to witness their wedding, which was absolutely beautiful. One of the days we were down there, my brother-in-law suggested a trip to Hollywood Studios—he wanted to take Karri on a rollercoaster because she'd never been on one before. I gave him a tepid half-smile and said, "Sure, sounds good." I didn't want to bring down the trip by mentioning my horrible memories from years ago. Well, I had so much anxiety driving there that you might have felt it if you had been within a few cars lengths from us on the highway.

When we got there I immediately saw one of the rides that I

hadn't been able to fit on all those years before. Right in front of the ride was the set of "tester seats", those are the actual seats for people to try to see if they can fit. I looked at my husband—he knew all about my stories of my previous visit, because he knows all.

He looked at me and said, "Babe, you're totally going to fit."

"No, I'm not," I said. "I'm too scared to even try."

He took my hand and led me to the seat. "Honey." He rubbed the top of my hand. "Yes, it's going to be okay. You're going to fit."

"No, I'm not. I just know it," I said as I looked around to see how many people could see what was going on here: fat girl is going to try and stuff her butt in the chair . . . again.

I slowly approached the stupid green chair that looked like the smallest chair in the entire world. There was just no way these legs and this butt were going to cram into it . . . there's just *no way*. Okay, the plan is I'm going to sit down really fast and then run away crying.

Well, I sat down and . . . holy hell and a baby goat, *I FIT!* I think my face looked like I'd just won the lottery. Boom! I was going on this ride. WEEEEEEEEEEEEEEE!

Another strange phenomenon from that recent trip was my lack of clothing. For my entire life, the more weight I put on, the more clothes I would put on to cover up. Who would want to see my body, my skin, and my pain when I could just cover it all up? Even during hot as balls summers I often layered on the clothes or wore jeans just to cover up my body. I think this was partially out of shame, and maybe something lingering from abuse, as well as just plain old wanting to hide.

This trip though, Karri wouldn't let me get away with that. She's always encouraging me to be bold with my style. She and I talked about our clothing for several weeks prior to the trip, trying to figure out what would be most comfortable for me to wear. Maybe maxi dresses? Capris? Bathing suits had to have skirts and maybe even a rash guard . . . whatever I could find to cover up, essentially. Then, right before we planned to leave, Swimsuits For All contacted me, asking me to shoot some selfies for them.

Me? *WHAT?!*

I know, I know, it was hard for me to believe too. But they really did. So when I talked to them they told me I could pick from any of the suits on their site. How awesome was that? I asked Karri and she said I *REALLY* needed a bikini, and one of the suits designed by Ashley Graham (total girl crush). GAH! Okay, maybe I could go a little crazy and try on one of those suits. What's the absolute worst that could happen? I would NEVER wear it in public, but I could at very least wear it in the bedroom for Mr. Wilder (More on that later, in chapter 12).

I took the leap and ordered some bathing suits I would have never, ever have imagined I could ever wear. Guess what? Yep, you know. You saw it on Instagram, right? Not only did I LOVE those suits, but I also sported them on the beautiful Florida beach with my husband. I did wear a sheer cover-up most of the time on my lower half, but this was a great, big, *huge* deal for me. I felt a tiny bit free and a tiny bit weird. Not like creepy weird, but more like the good/different sort of weird. A weird that might be good for me.

So, maybe I didn't need to be all covered up all the time. Maybe I was getting stronger inside and out. Maybe strong comes from little acts of bravery, starting from the outside in. When I look in the mirror these days, I don't always recognize myself. My doctor suggested taking lots of photos until the person in the mirror and the person I see in my head looks more like the person living in my body; it's an odd thing to try to come to grips with.

I've been one shape, one form, one very defined thing for so long that this new creature might take some time to get used to. She might take more time to appreciate. She might be a bit bolder, but also a bit more self-aware. She's learning to accept the new dips and arches of her body.

It's a good thing.

If you've lost a significant amount of weight, I recommend you give your body grace, and give yourself time. If this journey has taught me anything, it's that I really wasn't very kind to my body, and that it's very hard for me to ignore all of the very loud and negative things that my head is constantly yelling:

You're ugly.

You're still fat.

You have big feet.

Your nose is crooked.

Your loose, hanging skin is gross.

Your hips are too wide.

Those scars are so red, so deep.

It's funny how it is hard to write those things, but it is so easy to say them to myself. The fact is these voices, these lies, they *DO* leave marks. They do change us. This is why I've learned to talk back, to force my head and heart to hear the truth and not just believe the constant negative string of self-abuse radio that's always playing in the background. Now, I think: what would Jack say?

He'd say:

You're beautiful.

You're strong.

Your feet have carried you many, many miles.

Your nose, your eyes, your lips are perfect.

I love to touch your skin; it's so warm and soft.

Your hips are so curvy and sexy.

I don't even see those scars—I only see *you*.

How would your beloved talk about the things you most try to hide, that you're most critical of? My guess is your partner is less harsh on you than you are on yourself. Whatever the current state of your body, no matter where you are on the journey, be kind to yourself and to your body. Nothing is going to change overnight, but I think if we can turn the negative to the positive, the better we will feel, the stronger we will be and the happier we will be.

The old Jasinda is still here, but she's also different now. She's still blue moon, but maybe with a side of superwoman too!

PRO TIP: Always wear what makes you feel good, whatever it is. Just be you.

Chapter 5

RUNNING STILL SUCKS

"Do your best, one shot at a time, and then move on."
—Nancy Lopez

IF YOU STARTED RUNNING BECAUSE YOU READ MY BOOK, I PROBABLY owe you an apology. You probably hate me. You might even curse my name. I think I've even cursed my own name while running. Honestly it doesn't ever get better or easier, you just get stronger. It's hard for me, as a mom, to hide when I'm really not in the mood for our family runs. Usually my older daughter or my four-year-old son will start complaining first:

"We're going too far!"

"I hate running."

"This is stupid."

And most of the time I agree—it only takes about 5 minutes into my run before I'm questioning my own sanity. During my runs I'm wondering why I do this, when am I going to just drop, or should I call someone to pick me up so I don't have to run back? It's after I finish running, when I really feel strong, that I feel differently. And

that's as true now as when I first started running. I've never complet-
ed a run and wished I hadn't done it, or felt sorry that I got off the
couch and set out.

But I have had plenty of days when I wished I *had* run. There are
some days when I just feel off, or I can't get my mind and body to really get in the game and focus—those are the days when I wish I had
run. Running changes you even in small ways, step-by-step, block by
block, and mile by mile.

When my family first started doing 5K runs, we stuck to those
with level, even courses that would be easy with toddlers and stroll-
ers. I highly suggest you check out the route and course difficulty before signing up for a race; we learned this the hard way this summer
when I saw an advertisement for a local "Harvest Run."

Most of my readers know we are in northern Michigan in a very
agricultural area. A Harvest Run through orchards and vineyards—
sounds fun, right? Well, it's fun until you realize, halfway through,
that you're headed straight uphill for over a solid mile. These are the
times when you actually loathe running. When your legs and lungs
are burning, and you wish you could just lie down on the stupid hill
and let people use your motionless body as a speed bump.

Halfway through that run, I met up with a great group of ladies who felt the exact same way I did about that stupid hill. We all
kept grumbling about how we hated each and every step, stumbling
together over vines and rocks and holes. It was an experience that
might be best compared to a root canal performed on you by your
ex-husband. Okay, maybe not that bad, but pretty darn close. I honestly didn't think I was going to make it. The hilarious part was that
I remember thinking that my poor mother was behind me, and my
husband and three kids were somewhere ahead of me, so at least if I
died nearly everyone I loved would be close by.

That was actually the first run when anyone in our family received a medal. Jack finished first in his age division and my two oldest boys were first and second in theirs. Personally, I was just happy to finish. My mom thinks she did die somewhere around mile two and was forcibly reincarnated. I don't think I've ever heard her swear as much as she did that day. Didn't I tell you this would be loads of family fun? Just imagine how fun it was for my kids to hear grandma swearing. It was a blast, though. We were all so very proud of her as she crossed the finish line.

I know there's no way she would have made it to the end even a year ago, yet there we were, my mother and I . . . finishers! And there were my kids and husband, with medals around their necks, on a course that triathletes were using as training. WOW! Let me tell you how freaking amazing we felt at the end. We were glowing, bursting, laughing, and exhausted. This run wasn't just about health, this run was about strength. You have to be strong to scale a hill, people. That sort of workout is just no joke. As we were walking back to our van I kept thinking about how strong I felt, how I felt so many of my muscles as I was getting up those hills.

I guess you could say running was becoming a bit of a gateway drug for me. I wanted to feel more of that. I wondered just how many other muscles I might have hiding in there. As an obese person I had never really thought much about my muscles. They just weren't something that mattered. Any muscles that were in there wouldn't be seen, and as long as I could get from point A to point B, muscles didn't really matter.

Running forced me into a relationship with my muscles, and with my body. If you've carried lots of extra weight your whole life, this might be something you will experience, too. You'll start to notice that each time you run you can feel things happening in your body that you may have not felt before. You'll challenge yourself. Your body will meet you in these challenges.

Sometimes it is SO HARD, you'll probably want to quit the entire time. The coolest part for me during these family runs is that even though I may want to quit, I also want to keep going. I want to keeping going so I can get to the end and see the smiling faces of my kids and husband. Seeing them at the finish line, not only proud of themselves but also proud of *ME*. There's something about that you just can't describe. I don't run because of how it makes me look, I run because of how it makes me *feel*. Not just my physical body, but also my heart and mind, too. I believe this feeling comes from any physical activity when we're required to push ourselves, where our heart rate goes up and we have to join our bodies in the discipline of, "can't stop, won't stop."

I don't think there will ever be a time when I am going to pick running over shopping, chocolate, or Josh Cabernet Sauvignon, but nothing has ever given me long term joy like I've experienced from regular physical movement. The feelings that come from movement beyond what you think possible is nearly orgasmic. Don't believe me? Try it!

Today I did a new exercise program that my husband has been trying out for this book. We did 60 deadlifts, 60 weighted squats, 200 jumping jacks, 100 push-ups and 100 sit-ups on top of wogging a few miles. For most people that might not be so crazy, but for ME, for Jasinda Wilder, who weighed between 300 and 400 pounds her entire life, that's crazy-pants amazing. This poor body has been through so much. So many scary diagnoses. So much pain. That same body is now doing these things, and it feels amazing. It feels like I'm finally alive for the first time in my life!

I know that might sound crazy to some, but if you were a fat child like I was, a child that sat out in gym while watching the other kids running, climbing, and playing, then you understand.

Walking took me to wogging and then to running, and now it has lit a fire under me to see what other things my body might be able to do. You might be sitting there thinking that, yes, even if you've done a few 5Ks because Jasinda made you do it, there's still no way you could do any of the other things that are coming up in this book. You might even think I'm just straight-up crazy, but that is totally okay! You can think that before, during, and after trying this with us. I just want you to give me another 8 weeks.

Yes, running sucks, but it is also amazing too, right? Remember how you felt when you finished that first 5k? Let's keep at that and throw in some other things to tone, stretch, and add strength to your body. I believe you can do anything I can do. I believe you can probably even do better. You'll be running past me and lifting weights heavier than I can. I promise. In the next chapter we are going to talk about a simple plan to get you on the #WilderWay 2.0.

We've healed and cleaned our bodies, we've got ourselves moving, and now we're ready to get strong. You aren't in this alone. We are going to do this together. I know we can.

Get your strong on, girl.

Chapter 6

LIFTING WEIGHTS ALSO SUCKS

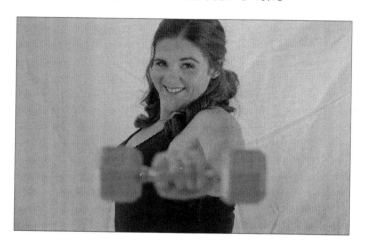

I ACTUALLY STARTED LIFTING WEIGHTS BEFORE MY HUSBAND DID. Don't let him tell you any differently. Not that it makes me an expert over him by any means, I just want the world to know that I was pumping up my muscles before Jack Wilder. Now, I know that some women may have weird feelings about lifting weights. Trust me, I totally understand why it's something you'd be afraid to try. You might be worried that you'll end up looking like Arnold Schwarzenegger, for example, but I *promise* that won't happen. That kind of specialized bodybuilding takes extreme dedication, endless hours in the gym, and an insane amount of work. This is not the kind of lifting I'm talking about.

Lifting, for me, is about toning my body and increasing the muscle mass around my bones so my body can be stronger. It's also good for me to have that extra muscle mass since I have an issue with bone density because of my nutritional disorder.

SIDE NOTE: I highly recommend you keep an eye on your bone density if you've had bypass, or any other sort of weight-loss surgery.

Let's talk about the benefits of picking up some weights:

- Performance—you will run faster and longer.
- It improves bone density.
- It promotes fat-free body mass.
- It increases the strength of connective tissue, muscles and tendons, which leads to improved motor performance and decreased injury risk.
- It improves your quality of life as you gain body confidence. Strength training will not only make you strong, but it will also help with managing your weight: weightlifting can help you burn fat, reduces your risk of diabetes, prevent back pain, and even help you fight depression.
- Increases HDL—High Density Lipoprotein (good cholesterol) and decrease LDL—Low Density Lipoprotein (bad cholesterol).
- Reduces risk of diabetes and insulin needs.
- Lowers risk of cardiovascular disease.
- Lowers high blood pressure.
- Lowers risk of breast cancer—reduces high estrogen levels linked to the disease.
- Decreases/minimizes risk of osteoporosis by building bone mass.
- Reduces symptoms of PMS (Premenstrual Syndrome)

- Reduces stress and anxiety.
- Decreases colds and illness.
- Mood boost.
- Better brain function.
- Building relationships (see chapter 12)

Okay, let's talk about a few of the benefits which are, I think, the most important, and are the main reasons I picked up weights in the first place. First, bone density—women have a higher chance of having issues with bone density than men at a rate of 6 to 1. More than half of all Caucasian women over 50 are estimated to have low bone mass, which means their bones are getting weaker, but they don't yet have osteoporosis. But, as we age, degeneration of the bones makes it easier for bones to break.

Special note to my author friends: living a sedentary lifestyle also puts us at higher risk for osteoporosis—any weight-bearing exercises and activities that promote balance and good posture are beneficial for your bones. Walking, running, jumping, dancing, and weightlifting are particularly helpful in fighting these bone density issues. I'm not saying any of this to scare you, but it's important to know, so we can be proactive with our health. If we continue to make small health changes and apply them to our lives, in ways that are doable and maintainable, we will have better long-term results. I love my author community and I want to see us all healthy and happy for a long time. We also have readers who might have similar tendencies to be sedentary. We all know how easy it is to get lost in a book and discover, eight hours later that we haven't moved for most of the day. Let's get off our butts and move!

I'm not one of those people who want to spend all day in the gym. I would much rather be in the kitchen, or playing with the kids or cuddled up on the couch with a good book. But, I have found that balance in all things is really important to our overall health and wellness.

As I talked about in *BIG GIRLS DO IT RUNNING*, I believe that our bodies are made to move. We are upright by design and when we aren't moving we are setting ourselves for health issues. Walking, wogging and running are all a great way to help your body and over-all health. Adding some weights will only add to that. When I started lifting I just wanted to add something easy on days when I couldn't find time to do a full walk/run. To be totally honest, I was thinking I could do some toning without actually breaking a sweat. Which, looking back, is patently ridiculous.

I would have the weights next to my desk and instead of farting around on Facebook when I needed to think in between paragraphs, I would pick up the kettlebell and just lift it in various ways I watched on YouTube and a few other websites. We will talk about these sites later on, but they were incredibly valuable to me when I was learning about different programs.

Also, it's important to note that I don't think you even need to go to a gym to be successful with a training program and, further-more, I think you can do this easily in almost any space and with minimal equipment. For example, my good friend Hugh only uses a few dumbbells for his program as he's sailing around the world. My mom is using simply some light weights and resistance bands, while Jack and I really like our small assembly of kettlebells.

Strength training is something everyone can do from home. Please don't think you can't become strong and fit if you have limited resources or are too busy to get to a gym. Just keep reading, because Jack and I have a beginner's guide coming that will make it easy for you to see and feel results in a relatively short amount of time.

After doing my kettlebell "breaks" in my office for a few months I decided I wanted to try a few more advanced routines. That is when I went and talked to Jack about having him work on a program with me. HUGE mistake, LOL. He was so excited about starting once I showed him a few videos. He actually started watching Russian kettlebell championships on his phone. I mean, who does that? Jack does—he's crazy. He then decided he wanted to start an intense program that was WAY over my level at that point. So I did what any loving wife who has a crazy hubby on a mission would do: I slept in on the mornings he did his training and kept to my beginner program.

This was actually God working in a mysterious way because now Jack and I have the unique experience of being at two very different levels trying to create a program that will work for everyone. I'm sure you all remember that I am really big on research, so while Jack was working on his high level kettlebell program, I was experimenting with all sorts of different popular exercise programs that combine free weights targeting specific areas with cardio.

Let me explain why I think this is important. First, I believe in getting your heart rate up. I like to run/walk in interval "bursts" as I've learned that's best for burning off that difficult fat. I like to do the same thing with my cardio. Had long-term cardio worked for me, my body would have looked quite a bit different when I was dancing four and five days a week as a teen. The truth is that 80% of your health comes from what you put in your body—your nutrition—and the other 20% is physical movement. That is why focusing on nutrition first is so very important—we have to get that going before we can start to change your shape and tone and strengthen your body.

I also want to point out here that I did take some heat in reviews for *BIG GIRLS DO IT RUNNING* because I ignored the "genetic" component to body shape and health. Here's my hard and honest truth about that: I don't think it plays as big a part as we've been told. In fact, I should go visit the endocrinologist who told me my issues were primarily genetic, because my body is now proof that genetics is not the whole story.

I think our physical shape, how we carry our weight, and how we digest food has more to do with the level of allergy we have to the sugar, chemicals, and other toxins currently in the majority of the food on our grocery store shelves. It might show itself in different ways in our bodies because we're all built differently but, trust me when I say you *can* be "skinny," or have a normal BMI, yet your body will still be riddled with the effects of these things. So if you want to call that genetics, fine, but it doesn't change the fact that the answer to these issues is the same. Once we get clean from these toxins and get moving, we can really start to target places to shape, tone, and build.

The program laid out later in this book is something that almost anyone can do with simple modifications. How will you know when you are ready? Well, you have to be brave enough to try. I think there is something to be said for timing. I do think you need to be in the right frame of mind for any program to be successful, but let me also say this: the time is *now*! Today is the day!

Here's the test I want to try right now. First, stand up. Yes, I'm assuming you are in the privacy of your own home. If you are listening on audio, or reading this while walking around your local grocery store, it might be best to try this when you get home—it will only take a few minutes and you can give me a one-star review if you die while attempting it. Okay, ready? Stand up and do 25 jumping jacks, 25 sit-ups, and 25 pushups. You can modify them however you want. I'll wait . . .

Still waiting . . .

Yes, I'm serious. #jasindamademedoit

Now, how do you feel? Do you feel horrible? Did you die? Sit and think about it for a few minutes if you have to. Feel your body. Does it feel good? Stronger? Do you think you could do a few more? Did you only do half? Listen, I've been at every stage of this. Remember when you wogged that first full minute and then the next day you did two? That is how we are going to get stronger too! One day at a time, one set at a time. If I can do this, you can, too. I'm the slowest of the slow and a mom of six with health issues a mile long. Just try this with me. Give me a bit more of your time. Listen to Jack. We are going to stay on this #WilderWay armed with new weapons. We've got armor and metal to go with our medal.

This is going to be fun, I promise!

PRO TIP : Don't hurt yourself. Start light and easy and build up. You have time to get into the heavier stuff. Small and gradual steps are the longest lasting.

STRONG AND HEALTHY MANTRA:

(To be said out loud, with strength and determination)

My body was created to be strong.
I was built to walk, run, move, jump, and dance.
My body is beautiful.
There is beauty in every single step of my journey.
I want to live a life of strength.
I'll allow myself to make mistakes.
I'll allow myself to be slow, to be weak, to be a starter.
I'll grow to become faster and stronger,
I'll grow to become a finisher.
Fear won't hold me back.
Family won't hold me back.
The voices in my head won't hold me back.
This is my time.
This is the day.
I *will* be strong.
I will walk, run, move, and dance.
My body will continue to be beautiful even when it changes.
I'll live a life of strength and beauty.
Each day is an opportunity to make better choices for my health
and strength.
Nothing will hold me back.
This is exactly the right time.
Today is the day I choose to find my strong.
One day at a time.
Slow, steady, and strong.

Chapter 7

HOW LONG DOES IT TAKE UNTIL WE ARRIVE AT FULL HEALTH?

"Believe me, the reward is not so great without the struggle."
—Wilma Rudolph

A QUESTION THAT COMES UP OFTEN IN MY FACEBOOK GROUP IS: How long does it take to lose all the weight we want? I wish there was an easy answer. In fact, I wish I could point to any part of this journey that has a simple answer.

First, each body is different. There are so many factors that dictate the rate your body will lose weight. I can tell you that, for most people, there is no rate fast enough. When you're in the midst of the journey it's going to seem like you're farther from the finish than you actually are. It always seems like you're never going to get there. But you *will*. I would even bet that when you get to your goal, when you get to that moment when you feel so good it brings you to tears, that's when you'll look back and be able to enjoy the journey and all the moments when you almost gave up, but didn't.

I remember about six months I was wogging with my family, and my husband turned around and snapped a photo of me. Here I was thinking I looked pretty darn healthy. I had already lost a considerable amount of weight and we had been doing a 5K race almost every month, so I was already starting to feel pretty strong. But that photo . . . ugh—that photo made me feel *horrible*. Although the top part of my body was starting to shrink, the bottom part of my body was holding on. My legs were rubbing together so badly I often had to cover them with powder and Body Glide.

To me, the photo showed a body that might never look normal. I was so upset that I wanted to give up. I cried my eyes out. Inside, I knew that the weight would eventually be shed from my legs, but it just wasn't quick enough. I was working so hard, I was always moving, and yet my mind was screaming all of my insecurities so loudly: I'll never be able to wear a "normal dress," my top will end up a size 10 and my bottom will still be a 20—these are the lies we tell ourselves. This is the ugly stepsister in my brain.

Now, when my husband takes a photo of me when we're all running together, my body actually looks pretty darn equal from top to bottom. Yes, my bottom half is still a bit larger, but I've learned to love it, especially with the help of my supermodel sisters like Ashley Graham, Iskra Lawrence, and Rosie Mercado. Have you seen those beautiful ladies? Wow!

When you feel like giving up, when it seems like nothing will work . . . HOLD ON! Just hang on a bit longer, because that's usually right when you have a breakthrough. This is the moment before you go down a size, or run your fastest mile, or drop that last stingy pound that was holding on as long as it could. Remember, when you feel like you're at your last straw, that's usually when your faith will be tested. But it's only going to make you stronger. This is when you get upgraded from contestant to champion, from competitor to warrior.

Don't give up on yourself, Mama! Fight! Talk back to the ugly stepsister in your head and let her know what's up. Get yourself singing some Taylor Swift, pick up your glittery guitar, shake it off, and bash that nasty bitch straight in the face. She's been talking enough during your life. Don't listen to her anymore.

But yet, I can hear you all groaning. Why can't there be some simple equation? If you know me, you know I hate doing math, but I'm going to offer you this as a baseline: each 25–50 lbs should take around a year to lose. Will some people lose faster? Yep! And will some lose more slowly? Absolutely! As I said before, this isn't a one-size-fits-all thing. I wish I could tell you exactly why some people will shed their excess weight faster than others, because gosh, I wish I was one of those people! I'm a sloth in the weight-loss game. Even now with only about 10–15 lbs more to lose to be really comfortable, I'm giving myself a solid year to do it. I don't want to eat into my muscle mass, and I want to tone, so I am giving myself and my body a full year to make that happen. If it doesn't happen within that year, I plan to grace myself with another six months.

Listen, this weight and health mess didn't happen in six days, six weeks, six months, or even six years. This is 36 years of wear and tear that I never want to deal with again. I'm determined to do it right. Maybe I've reached the ultimate level of stubbornness where I refuse to let a tiny setback claim victory over the war, and sisters, this *is* a war. It's a beautiful mess of a war, but it's still a war, and my body is crisscrossed with the scars to prove it. I'm sure many of you have those, too. It's okay, though, because one day we can all look at them together with pride, right? These are the stripes that have made me part of who I am today. These are the wounds that keep me going.

Don't hide them—be proud with me!

If you are six months or a year into this, as I'm sure many of you are, and you start to feel discouraged, please reach out for a reality check. Please ask a husband, friend, sister, or other source of support to remind you how far you've come. Pull out that iPhone and find a photo from six months or a year ago, get into your Instagram collage app, and put those photos side by side with the new you. Photos are often a good reality check because even when the scale doesn't show up for you, photos won't lie. You can even make that your screensaver as a reminder: every time you look at your phone know that you *are* making progress, that you *are* working towards better health.

I'll keep saying it, this is a marathon, not a sprint.

For some of us it might be one of those ultra marathons; I know that's how it feels for me. I feel like I'm rounding mile 40 or so, but I honestly wouldn't change a thing now. I know the time I am investing in myself now will be more time I'll get with my kids and grandkids later in my life. Each step spent wogging won't ever be wasted. Each healthy food choice I make is one that will make my body feel better.

I recently saw a meme that said something like "I'll never be on my deathbed wishing I hadn't had that cupcake." Well, I'm not so sure. As I watched my grandmother struggle with her diabetes, I'm pretty sure that no amount of heavenly cupcakes would have been worth her pain and suffering.

Do I think we should live a deprived life of treats? Heck, no! But I also know it's much easier to pick which kind of hard we want to live with: personally, I would rather spend a few extra bucks or minutes making a treat for my family that is going to be both nourishing and satisfying versus one slowly making us sick. I always try to make the best choices I can, moment by moment, day by day. These choices add up, and your family's health problems will slowly decrease, and you'll all start feeling petty damn good, and then suddenly having a firm handle on your health will become second nature.

I often hear a collective groan when I suggest that getting to a solid point with your health can take years, but let's be honest here:

most of us have been living the same way for years and years and years. We've been handed a life of food convenience, and now we're finally trying to swallow the price it came with. No, we won't change overnight. Some of us might have to keep trying over and over again. It might take two years of walking before we have the strength to run a full mile without stopping, but THAT IS OKAY! Any step toward a healthier lifestyle is a step worth taking. If you're one of those people who feel like you fail at everything, I totally understand. I'm one of you. The true test of success is hanging in there even when you feel like a total failure.

This isn't about a quick fix. This is about not giving up on yourself no matter what. No matter the stress, occasion, or disaster trying to pull you off your health plan. Yes, that stuff will happen, and you might even give in to some of those old temptations, but that's when you have to fight hardest, when you have to pick yourself up and make the best choices at the next meal. I believe in grace for our bodies, and for those of us with serious health and mental food issues, being kind to yourself and loving yourself is downright hard sometimes. The good news is that *you are not alone.*

Pick yourself up and wog on.

You *can* do this!

You are *worth* it.

From the CDC (Center for Disease Control): Effects of Obesity

- Risk of all causes of death are increased
- High blood pressure (Hypertension)
- High LDL cholesterol, low HDL cholesterol, or high levels of triglycerides (Dyslipidemia)
- **Type 2 diabetes**
- Coronary heart disease
- Stroke
- Gallbladder disease
- Osteoarthritis (a breakdown of cartilage and bone within a joint)
- Sleep apnea and breathing problems
- **Some cancers** (endometrial, breast, colon, kidney, gallbladder, and liver)
- **Low quality of life**
- Mental illnesses such as clinical depression, anxiety, and other mental disorders
- Physical pain and difficulty functioning

Chapter 8

I'VE GOT 99 PROBLEMS AND BURPEES ARE ABOUT 90 OF THEM.

"Champions keep playing until they get it right."
—Billie Jean King

LET ME TELL YOU A TINY SECRET: I'M NOT WONDER WOMAN. IN fact, most days I feel like a great big fuck-up. I think this is a pretty normal feeling for most American women these days.

There's just so much to do, right? We have to go to work, raise amazing kids, give our husbands the best sex, help at the kids' schools, volunteer at church, bake a cake for the fundraiser for abused animals, grocery shop (for me this activity alone takes a full day), keep your house looking like an HGTV crew could visit for an on-the-spot interview at any time, keep the kids clean . . . and now Jasinda wants me to find time to work out? Do something just for me?

Yeah, I know, I get it.

Our workouts need to be quick and dirty. I know time is precious, but I also know we can find time. Sometimes Jack and I get up before the kids to get a workout in. Sometimes we have to skip watching an episode of *Real Housewives*—I know, I know—just to make time for a workout. I personally prefer to do five workouts of

30–60 minutes each week. Sometimes we go hard with weights, and sometimes we just do a nice walk or run. There's no one-size-fits-all, *ever*, so do what makes you feel good.

The purpose of this book is two things: One, to encourage you. Two, to create a simple, no gym experience so strong that in 30 days you'll feel you can do this health and strength journey after all. I really think sometimes it just takes someone telling you that you *can* to make all the difference.

Here are some time tricks I've found that help with my busy life; I'm going to call them #WilderWay fitness hacks.

- Walk whenever you can.
- If you're going to the store, park in the farthest spot from the door, not the closest.
- Make a goal of doing some sort of squat or lunge each time you go to the bathroom—usually I try to do at least 10 of something. And, yes, you might look silly if someone catches you, but just think about how freaking amazing that butt is going to look!
- Make exercise a family activity—maybe you have a backyard where you can do some jumping jacks and sit-up challenges with your kids, or just move the couch and coffee table out of the way, whatever it takes!
- When you carry your kids to bed, try to use your muscles and fully engage your body.

I know these things seem very minor but they add up. And hey—have you signed up for your next 5K?

Here are a few other easy ideas:
- Speed-walk or power-lunge through the kitchen.
- Get down on the floor and play with the kids.

- Carry heavy things like groceries and lift them as you carry them inside.
- Flex those glute muscles regularly.
- Plank—I try to do three reps (repetitions) of one minute each before I shower.
- 50 sit-ups/pushups before bed (this is especially fun with wine and a friend).
- Walk the dog.
- Squat!
- Join a team! My husband really enjoyed subbing for an adult softball team over the summer.
- Get a wearable movement tracker and challenge your colleagues, friends, and/or family to movement goals.
- Run or walk while the kids are at dance or sport practice—I found that walking the track while my son was at football practice was a great way to kill two birds with one stone.

Remember, any movement counts. It's best to try and get that heart rate up periodically even if you need to take breaks. Heck, even seasoned and conditioned athletes take breaks. It's Okay!

Sometimes, when my husband tells me about our next day's workout, my first response is: "no freaking way I can do that!" There are always going to be days like that, but as long as you make an effort each day, be proud of yourself. I also think it's super helpful to have a friend, husband, wife, or child to work out with. Jack or Nanny Karri (now, my sister-in-law) are my usual workout partners. They're always so encouraging, and they push me to keep going when I want to give up . . . which is pretty much every set.

Here's the thing, though: part of me wants to tell you that you should only do things that are fun and that you enjoy, but I've learned that some workouts—which sounded totally horrible, painful, and awful—are the ones I feel the most badass about finishing. The days I felt like there was no way I could ever do the workout we had planned are the days I ended up feeling the strongest.

So I actually want to encourage you to try the things you think you could never do, things that make you feel a big uncomfortable, things that might make a mom of six pee on herself—cue the commercial for THINX active underwear . . . I'm just being honest, these things do happen when you're jumping around. It's okay!

And here's my other piece of advice: Don't worry if you never get the "perfect" form. If you have to modify a move, that's okay too! Just do it the best you can. Often we have a vision in our heads that includes us needing to be perfect at something to be able to participate. This is silly, Momma! You're a beginner at most of these things. Just ask Jack about my burpees!

Early on in our hard and fast, quick and dirty training, Jack tried to tell me we were going to do 50 burpees. Which didn't sound too difficult until I actually tried to complete *one* freaking burpee. I swear, those damn things were invented by the devil himself. Sometimes my body revolts so hard that I actually have to scrape myself off of the floor. Lying on the ground and then getting up is hard enough 50 times in a row *without* having to actually jump at the top of the movement.

So, I modified and slowed down and kept struggling until the next time we did them they were a tiny bit easier. I say "tiny bit" because I believe nothing on the whole earth will ever make burpees easy. I'll never like them, but I'm never going to stop doing them either.

Important Note: I'll never, *ever,* let anyone but my husband and Karri ever see me attempt to do them . . . it's just a hot mess that no one needs to see.

Which brings up another topic I want to elaborate on: the gym, the public, and exercise. I do think when you're starting out it's really important for you to feel comfortable doing some of these basic moves without being watched or judged. We all remember the Playboy Bunny making fun of grandma, right? Not that this will happen to us, but I know people who won't step into a gym because they're worried about being judged or laughed at. I had gym memberships at some of my heaviest weights and, honestly, I do feel sometimes having eyes on me made things more difficult, but that's something you really need to decide for yourself.

I think you should work out whenever and wherever work for you. For us, the home gym is perfect. We use very minimal equipment, and most of it is relatively inexpensive and doesn't take up much space. You can check out places like Rogue fitness (www.roguefitness.com) which has great packages for starter garage/home gyms.

Here are some of my favorite starter home gym must-haves (also check your local sports resale store, or Craigslist for great deals on these):

- A step for deep lunges and power jumps.
- A few sets of free weights or kettlebells: 5 lb, 10 lb and 15 lb are a great start. If you want to invest in a really great set, we love the Bowflex adjustable dumbbells—you can find these on Amazon for about $250 per pair; they adjust from 5 lb all the way up to 52.5 lb!
- A jump rope.
- A yoga mat.
- Exercise stability ball—I like the extra big ones.
- A quality weight bench.

- Jack and I both love using an Olympic barbell, but you can often use dumbbells for similar movements, so I suggest getting those or kettlebells first because you can get a lot of use out of a good set of those.
- A doorway pull-up bar is also nice to have.
- A treadmill for when the weather keeps you indoors.

And that's really all you need to get started. We built our basement home gym slowly, so please don't feel like you need all of these things right off the bat in order to be successful.

Most of the work I do is with my 15 or 20 lb kettlebells and my mat. There's so much you can do to work your body with minimal equipment, and even a lot you can do without any equipment at all—Jack will talk more about bodyweight exercises in his chapter.

But, don't I need a trainer to do these things?

Actually, I don't think you do. There are so many great videos online, lots of challenge programs and wonderful tutorials that make it easy to work out on your own. We do research a lot, but that's part of how our writers' minds work.

I think with some basic movements and equipment, and your wogging, you can achieve some wonderful success at home. Let's be honest here: I don't think most of us are planning on entering a bikini contest anytime soon. We just want to have good health and increased physical strength so we can run with the kids and keep up with the basic activities of life without being fatigued and out of breath.

If you *are* looking to compete or really build lots of muscles, you might need a trainer or more advanced equipment and techniques, but for basic improvement in your physical ability and strength, what Jack and I are going to lay out is a great place to start. Once you get started you'll probably want to keep going; I know this is what happened with Jack and me. It started with a 30-day challenge we did together and now we feel weird if we aren't doing something to increase the challenge in our workouts. The key, and the hardest part, is just getting started. Let's get moving!

Jasinda's Quick and Dirty 30 Days to a Fitter, Stronger You, for Beginners: Wilder Way 2.0

(Don't forget to take a before photo! I want to see them!)
*Jack has some intermediate and advanced exercises plans coming later on, don't worry!

1. Warm up: One mile of walking/wogging or running as fast as you can. It's okay to stop as needed, just push yourself and get that heart rate up.
2. Pick **any three or four** of these basic strength movements and rotate daily. Yes, you can modify these if needed! They don't have to be perfect, just get 'em done! Set a timer and see how fast you can do the three movements, and try to beat your best times. This is my go-to workout plan. It doesn't get old because I just keep changing up the order I do them in and which movements I pick. I love these because they get the heart rate up and they don't take long. I also record daily what combo I do and the time it takes me to do the sets. If I want to challenge myself I will add weights to some of these and then do some sprint bursting to end my workout. I don't have time to work out for hours and this will give me great results in a short amount of time. If these numbers start to feel too easy and you are getting through the workout

really fast, just add more sets or increase the number you are doing for each exercise.

- 25 jumping jacks
- 20 pushups or sit-ups
- 1-minute plank—30 second side planks are fine too! These are great for strengthening your core.
- 12 lunges to the back or side (6 on each leg)
- 15 squats or 10 jump squats
- 10 straight leg lifts
- 1-minute wall sit
- 30 second sprints
- 25 high knees
- 15 hip thrusts
- 20 butterfly kicks
- 20 mountain climbers (10 each leg)
- 1 minute of jumping rope

You can swear at me if you want, but I want you to try and run at top speed for at least a half mile for bonus points.

I promise, after 30 days of doing this 4–5 times each week, you're going to see results and want more. So grab a friend and get started! We've got more exercises and workout plans coming and we want you ready for them! Challenge each other and try to have fun with it. Time yourself and keep track. We try to improve our times and always play some fun music in the background—you know we stop for awesome dance breaks!

PRO TIP: bodybuilding.com and breakingmuscle.com are our go-to websites for fitness videos, sample workouts, and tips. The Breaking

Muscle website has the most comprehensive video library on kettle-bell moves anywhere. AIM Fitness Networks and the WORKOUT app are both great resources for workouts and videos.

Chapter 9

#WILDERWAY EVOLUTION

Stop Being Hungry on White Plate Day and EAT!

As Jack and I continued on our health journey, we started to feel things over and over again that had me tweaking our plan. One of the things that really occurred to us on white plate days—I say "days" because you'll see as we go on that we're going to adjust the plan into full black and white days for most of the week—we were ALWAYS hungrier on white plate days.

Hungry to the point where I was thinking about food WAY too much. It was starting to feel like a diet again, and I *hated* that. In fact, it would sometimes send me into a panic. I would be on the way to pick up the kids and I'd have to pull over to eat nuts, or break out my emergency protein bar.

This was *only* happening on the days we worked out more, which were our white plate days because we knew we needed the extra carbs for workout and recovery. Jack satisfied his hunger by snacking pretty much all day, but I personally didn't want to do that. It felt good to be at a place where I wasn't ruled by food and I didn't want to go back to that slavery. So, I started using myself, Nanny

Karri, and my mom as guinea pigs to try and tweak certain things. The great thing is that the three of us represent most age groups and health issues, so I knew most of my bases were covered.

What you'll read below is the result of about six months of constant tweaks and adjustments to the original Wilder Way—you'll notice it really isn't a huge change from the original plan. Starting out, I think it's best to begin carb cycling meal by meal, since it's honestly easier for most people. As you get into the flow of carb cycling it will become second nature—for me, it's just a way of life, now.

I'm guessing many of you might feel like you're still learning about your body, its responses to different fuels, and reactions to cycling. Guess what? I am too! It's amazing to me what I'm still learning, and how I'm still surprised by the things my body can do when I take care of it and fuel it properly.

When your body tells you something, *listen*; when you're hungry, *eat*.

I don't think our body makes mistakes—I believe our bodies are divinely crafted and perfectly made, and if we just listen to what our bodies are telling us, we'll be much better off. The body WANTS to heal. So when you're doing more intense exercise and burning more calories, and especially when you're lifting weights, you really need to eat more, and eat more frequently. This not only makes sense logically, but I've felt it and I've seen the evidence in my own body.

I also know my body likes a steady routine in which I can consistently eat foods that keep me happy, healthy, and satisfied. As you already know, I refuse to be unsatisfied, and I hate feeling like I'm missing out on something; I LOVE FOOD!

The minor changes to the Wilder Way plan made it not only easy, but I felt even more satisfied and happy knowing which fuel types we would be having each day. This also opened me up to types of foods I had been scared of before . . . we're eating way more veggies, even my husband! YAY JACK! I make sure we get greens at every single meal. Yes, this took some getting used to, but the results we saw from doing this has been huge. I'm totally on Team Kale!

Below are two options for a typical week in terms of food and exercise.

THE WILDER WAY 2.0—OPTION #1

HIGH OCTANE FUEL, HEAVY TONE, HOT SCULPT

MONDAY: (WHITE PLATE DAY)

HEAVY WORKOUT—40 min of weight lifting and cardio.

Three meals *and* three snacks—CARBS AND PROTEINS in each meal and snack.

Little to no fats at all!

TUESDAY: (WHITE PLATE DAY)

HEAVY WORKOUT—40 min of weight lifting and cardio.

Three meals *and* three snacks—CARBS AND PROTEINS in each meal and snack.

Little to no fats at all!

WEDNESDAY: (BLACK PLATE DAY)

LIGHT WORKOUT—30 min of dancing or light core work, little to no weight lifting.

Three meals and *two* snacks—FATS AND PROTEINS in each meal and snack.

Low carbs all day!

THURSDAY: (WHITE PLATE DAY)

HEAVY WORKOUT—40 min of weight lifting and cardio.

Three meals *and* three snacks—CARBS AND PROTEINS in each meal and snack.

Little to no fats at all!

FRIDAY: (WHITE PLATE DAY)

HEAVY WORKOUT—40 min of weight lifting and cardio.

Three meals *and* three snacks—CARBS AND PROTEINS in each meal and snack.

Little to no fats at all!

SATURDAY: (BLACK PLATE DAY)

LIGHT WORKOUT—run or walk with family, or dance videos for easy and fun cardio.

Three meals and two snacks—FATS AND PROTEINS in each meal and snack.

Low carbs all day!

SUNDAY: (GRAY ALL DAY!) Yes! PTL!

We use Sunday as what most bodybuilders would call a "refeed." I have to say, this was my favorite part of the Wilder Way 2.0 tweaks. Now you can have your regular French Toast with Ezekiel or other sprouted bread, or toast with your eggs. You can have a burger on a sprouted bun, or nachos with blue corn chips *and* CHEESE AND SOUR CREAM! Can you tell how excited I am about this? Yes, it really is exciting.

THE WILDER WAY 2.0—OPTION #2

LOWER OCTANE FUEL, LIGHT TONE

MONDAY: (WHITE PLATE DAY)

HEAVY WORKOUT—40 min of weight lifting and cardio.

Three meals and three snacks—CARBS AND PROTEINS in each meal and snack.

Little to no fats at all!

TUESDAY: (BLACK PLATE DAY)

LIGHT WORKOUT—30 min of a dance video or light core work, very little or no lifting.

Three meals and two snacks—FATS AND PROTEINS in each meal and snack.

VERY LOW CARBS!

WEDNESDAY: (BLACK PLATE DAY)

LIGHT WORKOUT—30 min of a dance video or light core work, very little or no lifting.

Three meals and two snacks—FATS AND PROTEINS in each meal and snack.

VERY LOW CARBS!

THURSDAY: (WHITE PLATE DAY)

HEAVY WORKOUT—40 min of weight lifting and cardio.

Three meals and three snacks—CARBS AND PROTEINS in each meal and snack.

Little to no fats at all!

FRIDAY: (BLACK PLATE DAY)

LIGHT WORKOUT—30 min of a dance video or light core work, very little or no lifting.

Three meals and two snacks—FATS AND PROTEINS in each meal and snack.

VERY LOW CARBS!

SATURDAY: (BLACK PLATE DAY)

LIGHT WORKOUT—run or walk with family, or a dance videos for easy and fun cardio.

Three meals and two snacks—FATS AND PROTEINS in each meal and snack.

VERY LOW CARBS!

SUNDAY: (GRAY ALL DAY!) Yes! PTL!

We use Sunday as what most bodybuilders would call a "refeed." Now, this was my favorite part of the Wilder Way 2.0 tweaks. Now you can have your regular French Toast with Ezekiel or other sprouted break or toast with your eggs. You can have a burger on a sprouted bun, or nachos on blue corn chips WITH CHEESE AND SOUR CREAM! Can you tell how excited I am about that? Yes, it's just that exciting.

In my testing, I found some people, because of health issues, were unable to lift weights or do high-intensity aerobics. In those cases, there might be too many carbs in Option #1 for them to burn off. Lower carbs might also work better for those who are just more carb-sensitive, too.

If you can, I would suggest trying Option #1 for a week and

then make a decision based on how you feel. I should point out that it can take a few weeks before you really get into the groove and for your body to get on board, so give yourself some time, but also know you have options. Some people feel best when rotating Option #1 and Option #2—meaning two weeks of Option #1 and two weeks of Option #2 each month. That is fine too! When you want to mix things up, you can try these options and then go back to the original plan from BGDIR.

This is meant to be very flexible and can and should be adjusted to fit what works for *you*. We are currently loving Option #1 as we are trying to increase our muscles and strength, but we will absolutely switch things up when we need to. Do what works for you and make this fun! I've noticed that I've gone from dreading white plate meal days to loving them. I've relearned to enjoy the wonderful and comforting foods that are carbs—more on that in the next chapter.

Another easy #WilderWay 2.0 modification is alternating black and white days so that you are high carb one day and low carb the next and then back up to high carb. This works well if you're only getting in heavy workouts every other day. Remember, this plan can be tailored to fit any lifestyle at any pace. Do what works for you and listen to your body!

I'll have lots of ideas for you coming up in regards to your meals and snacks, so don't worry . . . just keep reading. I know you can do this! If you're reading this and have no clue what I'm talking about when I say white and black plates, please go back and review *BIG GIRLS DO IT RUNNING*. It's really important to understand the different plate combinations first, one day at a time and one meal at a time.

PRO TIP: Always keep your food list and plate graphics handy; visit www.biggirlsdoitrunning and print out several. I have them in my purse and on the counter, because even the pros can use a reminder now and then.

Chapter 10

CARBS ARE NOT EVIL MONSTERS!

*"Foods high in **carbohydrates** are an important part of a healthy diet. **Carbohydrates** provide the body with glucose, which is converted to energy used to support bodily functions and physical activity."*
—Harvard.edu

OKAY FRIENDS, WE'VE TALKED ABOUT THIS *AD NAUSEAM*, BUT I think it's REALLY important, so we are going to go over it again. The things I call "healthy carbs" are not your enemy—they were designed to help your body. When used correctly, carbs will make your body stronger, will give you more energy, and will help you feel ready to run!

Here's my list of healthy carb options (WHITE PLATES):

- Sprouted bread: Ezekiel, Silver Hills, Pepperidge Farms, Aldi Brand
- Sprouted or whole wheat tortillas
- Cereal: Ezekiel, Uncle Sam Original
- Blue, baked corn chips
- Old Fashioned Oats
- Apples (green have lower glycemic impact)

- Banana
- Popcorn (minus butter or oil)
- Quinoa
- Rice (brown or sprouted)
- Brown rice pasta
- Beans
- Hummus
- Lentils
- Carrots
- Sweet potato
- Butternut squash
- other fruits depending on your tolerance

Now, let's just be honest about this . . . many of us grew up in a time when low carb and/or low fat diets were popular fads. It's only normal, then, that many of us are afraid to load up on carbs, but not all carbs are created equal. The carbs I listed above won't hurt you, and they will actually help you gain strength and be more energetic. They aren't the nasty, highly-processed carbs of our youth. The carbs on my list are *superfoods*. They give us energy and help us find our strong.

When we started the *BIG GIRLS DO IT RUNNING* Facebook group I received message after message after message about carbs. This is one of the biggest issues most women of my generation have in terms of health and nutrition. In fact, the current paleo trend is primarily a knee-jerk response to our current fear of carbs.

I would *never* eat any of those nasty, evil, processed, fake food-like-product carbs, but that doesn't mean we need to toss out *all* of the foods in this group. When you look at the foods God created for us to enjoy, each one plays a very important part in our overall nutrition, so let's allow our bodies to enjoy these comfort foods in a healthy, nourishing way.

When I say you need to eat lots of these healthy carbs on White Plate days, what exactly does that mean? Well, it means that you really need to focus on eating a lot of healthy carbs on those days, and not just dip a toe into the carb pool. I remember when we first started the first 8-week Wilder Way challenge someone sent me a photo of their White Plate dinner, and I think it had one tiny spoonful of rice. That's not going to work, people! We need to have a reasonable portion of carbs for this regimen to be effective. Three or four grains of rice just isn't sufficient. Sorry!

Below is an example of a pretty typical White Plate day for us:

WHITE PLATE DAY (Jasinda's day of meals and snacks—eating approximately every two hours):

BREAKFAST: Old Fashioned Oats with yogurt and berries

BREAKFAST SNACK: Chocolate Jay Robb shake with ½ a frozen banana and oats.

LUNCH: Egg salad sandwich on sprouted bread made with boiled egg whites only. Spinach and seasoning to taste. (FLAVORGOD seasoning is great for this)

LUNCH SNACK: carrots and bell peppers, ranch dip (made with plain Greek yogurt and FLAVORGOD ranch seasoning), turkey slices (natural without nitrates), and a few apple slices

DINNER: Ground turkey and brown rice pasta spaghetti with salad

DINNER SNACK: Cottage cheese with a few peach slices or blueberries and some Ezekiel cereal for crunch—1 cup of fat-free cottage cheese, a cup of fruit, and half a cup of Ezekiel almond cereal. I also add some sweetener or even some vanilla Jay Robb protein powder if I want to add more protein too. I LOVE this snack.

Please note that when I say "snack" I'm not messing around. Yes, this is a *big* snack, but it's really great for my body, and I'm a big girl. You don't have to eat this much, but I want you to see that I'm not eating a tiny portion of carbs here. Your body will adjust to the amount of food you're eating, to the point that you'll find yourself getting hungry every two hours, especially on days when you've done a heavy workout. I'm eating a FULL serving of delicious and healthy carbs every time I eat . . . and this is a lot of carbs!

I know this seems like A LOT of food—because it is! When you're lifting and doing high-intensity cardio, your body will burn these fuels very quickly. Your body is telling you that it requires more fuel. I've found on days like these that I'm very satisfied and full and I see wonderful results, especially in terms of toning and burning fat.

When Jack and I really got into the groove with this 2.0 plan, we both saw changes in the way our clothes fit every 2-3 weeks. This was about twice as fast as we had seen before we increased the dietary carbs and before we started strength training. Muscle mass increased much faster, and fat burned off faster, and I saw my running times and endurance get much better. The other thing that Jack and I both noticed was that we slept better too—when you spend the day burning fat, for some reason your body will rest more easily.

We also increase our water intake on these days; we both try to drink at least half a gallon of water a day, if not a full gallon. On top of maintaining proper hydration, water is extremely important in flushing out your body's toxins, so don't forget about getting lots of water even when you feel full from eating. Water is critical to keep your body functioning properly. Keep your fluids close by!

PRO TIP: I have my 27 oz Swell bottle with me at all times. If I'm at home, it's on my desk, my bedside, or on a nearby table. When

I'm in my car, it's in the cup holder, at church it's in my purse, and at the grocery store it's in the cart. I try to fill and drink the whole thing four times each day. Now, this does mean I pee a lot, but I'm healthy and I think my body thanks me for the hydration. Heck, it might even be filling up some of my wrinkles. I'm getting close to 40, people; I need all the help I can get!

Chapter 11

NO MORE STALLS!

Jumpstart and Reset 2.0

THIS CHAPTER IS PROBABLY GOING TO BE A BIT CONTROVERSIAL, but I've decided I'm okay with that. Listen friends, I'm sharing with you what has worked for me, and for those who have tried this plan with me. Will it work for *everyone*? I honestly doubt it, but since I've opened this big can of worms I think it's important not to leave out any part of my journey and story.

There was a stretch of about two months when my weight loss was completely stalled. I think this was because of two things: A) I dramatically increased my physical activity and my body was trying to adjust, and B) my body just needed time to regroup.

I went through all my other tried-and-true stall-busters, and literally nothing was working. If I said I wasn't discouraged I'd be lying, because I was. Even though I knew my body would eventually resume the downward trend, it was difficult to wait for physical, tangible results.

Finally, after much frustrating experimentation, I found something that worked. Subsequently, I've seen it work for some of my beta readers who were experiencing similarly frustrating stalls. What is that something? It is a 1–3 Day Fast.

Yes, I know . . . I never liked the idea of fasting, but this really isn't a true fast, more of a cleanse and a temporary plan modification. This isn't something I would do all of the time, and by the end of day three I'm usually craving meat so badly I would almost go outside and find one of my chickens . . . JUST KIDDING!

It is often not easy—but I also think fasting can be very healthy and effective. My thoughts on this have been borne out by several recent books and studies that show that doing this sort of cleanse or "fast" is great for you.

As always, before making any significant changes to your health and wellness plan, I suggest you consult with your doctor and talk about whether it is right for you.

Please remember, you could just be slowed down but not totally stalled. If this is the case you *won't* need to do this at all. The loss of a half-pound or pound—or even as much as two pounds per week—is perfect. Give your body time and grace. You're doing great!*

Jasinda's STALL-BUSTER Plan

This dietary adjustment can be done for 1–3 days. I usually go back to a BLACK PLATE day after this because my body will really need the fats.

Rules:
- As little dairy as possible, none at all if you can manage it.
- No meat of any kind.
- As many veggies as possible.

- Three "meals" and at least one snack every day. Most of the items on your plate are going to be totally neutral, with a few exceptions.

Example of a typical day in the stall-buster cycle:

BREAKFAST: Super veggie shake with Jay Robb protein powder and collagen, and one or two pieces of spouted bread with minimal almond butter

LUNCH: Large salad of kale and spinach with veggies, hemp seeds, nutritional yeast, non-dairy dressing, and FLAVORGOD seasoning, plus two Wasa crackers with Laughing Cow cheese on the side; sometimes I'll add some egg whites as a side or add them into my salad. Mini smoothie of Jay Robb protein powder, almond milk or water, and berries.

SNACK: a nice big handful of almonds.

DINNER: Large salad with rice or another grain on the side, and a chocolate, okra (yes, I said okra) and PB smoothie.

PLEASE NOTE: I do not suggest eating this way beyond the three days of the stall-buster. I don't think it is maintainable long-term, and it should *only* be used in the plan when you are in a long-term stall, or you feel like you've been "off the wagon" and need a cleanse or fast to heal your body before starting back into the program. This is a tool that I've also found works really well after a day where I've "celebrated" a little too much and I'm feeling really heavy or bloated . . . you know, those days when you don't feel like eating, but you know you need to.

The stall-buster can be used for just one meal or one day. This year I did this for breakfast and lunch after Thanksgiving, and it really helped me to get back into the gym. You'll have lots of energy from the goodness in the all the greens and grains.

Just make sure you keep focusing on how your body is feeling. The longer I've been on the #WilderWay, the easier it is for me to listen to what my body needs. I often find myself crave my super veggie shakes loaded with kale, spinach, okra, and green apple. I can really tell when my body needs those extra nutrients.

It's also important to repeat, as I said in *BIG GIRLS DO IT RUNNING*, that you still need to eat food at each meal. I don't believe in replacing a meal with just a shake. Make sure you're crunching and munching on something to keep your metabolism moving and your body digesting normally—as it was created to do.

The great thing about this mini-reset is that I don't see the upward trending people often saw in earlier results of the program. This seems to really support the steady downward trend.

I also think it's a great idea to be journaling—keep track of how your body feels during these new days. Tune into your body and treat it right.

Chapter 12

SEXY TIMES WITH YOUR NEW BODY

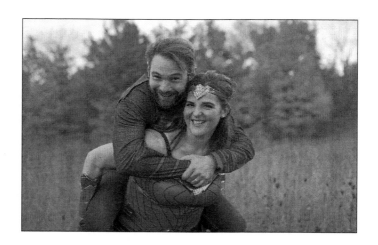

Jasinda says:

I'M ABOUT TO TELL YOU SOMETHING TOTALLY NUTS. CRAZY! Like, headline worthy. I should probably even change the title of this book to reflect the craziness I'm about to lay out in this book. Let me first say, however, that it probably shouldn't come as a shock to anyone at this point that my husband and I have A LOT of sex. We have lots of kids, we write romance, we are both super good-looking . . . AMIRIGHT?! Okay, don't answer that!

Regardless, we love each other so much and we probably look like silly, horny teenagers much of the time when we're out in public. I'm okay with it. Our physical relationship has always been GREAT! I also tell my husband that even when I think it couldn't get any better, I'm always surprised to find out it does. #Blessed!

As I'm trying to get my balls together to really let this out, just remember that I do write pretty graphic stuff. ***Mom, please stop reading.***

So, even though we've always had a wonderful and successful sex life with plenty of orgasms to go around, I have to admit I never had a freaking clue where my G-spot was. Over thirty-five years old and I was starting to think my G-spot was something like the Bermuda triangle, or Santa, or the Easter bunny. Or maybe I was just born without one? Was that even possible? I can't be the only one who has ever thought that.

Also important to point out is that Jack and I have tried nearly every possible position allowable by gravity. But no position, no search and rescue mission, and no deep dive session ever made it possible to find the darn thing. Well, guess what? As I continued to lose weight something incredible happened!

I FOUND IT!

I think the excess stomach weight had somehow made it near impossible to ever be in a positon to access it. Why am I telling you this rather personal tidbit? Well, here's why: good health reveals all sorts of hidden treasures! Having lots of energy, muscles, and strength will only make your sex life better. Yes, I still struggle sometimes with the parts of my body that are scarred, and/or loose with skin but overall, the abilities of my body have only continued to improve. This will happen for you, too. I promise, friends.

One thing that Jack and I are always amazed by is that even after a long day, putting the kids to bed, and making time for a workout, we still have the energy, stamina, and even the need to partake in some marital time. Yes, we usually enjoy a nice glass of Cabernet first, but even after the regular stress of six kids, a farm, and this crazy publishing business and all that comes with it, we are still ready, willing, and able. It surprises us, too! I think working out with your husband will only make your marriage and sex life stronger and more enjoyable. Having a lot of good sex is even a bonus workout, if you ask me. So, don't be afraid to get it on and get those extra bonus points for just having fun!

Jack says:

There's been an enormous number of benefits to my increased healthiness since starting the #WilderWay. As my wife has stated several times already, both in this book and the first one, when you cut out the evil, not-food nastiness that is 80% of the products on the grocery store shelves, your body just . . . works better in every way. Increased energy, strength, motivation, endurance . . . and stamina.

As Jasinda said, we've always had intense sexual chemistry, and our sex life has always been consistently active and amazing. And then we cut out sugar and processed food-like products (notice we aren't calling any of that stuff "food," because it's NOT FOOD!), and our sex life got better. Our bodies were operating more smoothly, reaching closer to peak capacity. The chemistry between us improved, our desire for each other increased, and our—*ahem*—performance improved.

That was phase one of Operation Hotter Wilder Sex.

Phase two happened when we increased our carb load a bit and started getting serious about strength training through bodyweight and resistance workouts—more on those from me later on. We got stronger, leaner, more powerful, and had better endurance. Guess what? Sex got EVEN BETTER! I could support my weight on my arms for longer, and because my core was stronger, certain . . . errr . . . movements, shall we say, were easier and could be performed for longer and more powerfully. Other-than-missionary positions were easier. My sheer physical stamina increased, and my sexual stamina—the length of time I could hold out—improved. And finally, our physical shapes were different. We both had less belly in the way, which meant the way we fit together changed . . . for the better.

Once we detoxed from the poisons we were eating, and then got our metabolisms pumping and our muscles enlarging and that fat burning away, our bodies just worked better from top to bottom, inside and out. Those toxins were clogging up and slowing down everything from our brains to our bowels, metabolisms to muscle mass, sensory input to sexuality. Clear all that up, and the perfectly-designed machine that is the human body suddenly just *works*. It's amazing, honestly.

There's another element to this other than the physical. Mentally, emotionally, psychologically, we felt better about ourselves, and I think it's no surprise to anyone when I say that self-image and confidence are HUGE factors in sexual performance for both men and women—and if any dude says otherwise, he's lyin'.

If you don't feel like you *look* good, or if you just don't *feel* good, then your sexual desire and performance will suffer. Conversely, you might find that when you shed those extra pounds and reduce your clothing sizes you discover your muscles. You start to enjoy running and working out, you feel better about how you look, and you just feel better, and so . . . sex improves.

Before we started this journey, I was what you'd call skinny-fat. Looking at me, you wouldn't have called me overweight, but the weight I did carry was all soft, doughy fat with small, weak muscles. My metabolism was clogged up and I had no drive, no motivation to move. Sound familiar? Yeah, I thought so. Then I started eating what my wife told me to eat, in the order she told me to eat it, and I suddenly had energy I needed to burn, which meant I wanted sex more and was better at it. Which meant my wife enjoyed it more, which meant she wanted it more, which meant I, in turn, wanted it *even* more, and wanted to be stronger and healthier and have more endurance and stamina so I could be even better at it . . . see how it all works together?

Also, finding her G-spot was mind-blowing, for both of us. #G-spotFTW

PRO TIP: Buy a Womanizer Pro40 (You can thank me later; yes, it's worth every penny.)

Chapter 13

BE PICKY AND PRIORITIZE YOUR PROTEIN

I F YOU ASK MY HUSBAND, HE'LL TELL YOU I'M SOMEWHAT OBSESSED with all things non-fiction; I *devour* non-fiction books. I love memoirs, cookbooks, documentaries, and health and fitness books. I usually read a few each week, even during busy weeks . . . which is all of them. My kitchen is overflowing with cookbooks, and even though most of my other books end up on my eReader, I just *have* to have my big, colorful and juicy cookbooks; they're stacked all over my kitchen and in my cupboards.

SIDE NOTE: Doing a beautiful, sexy cookbook is on my bucket list, so if you're a publisher reading this and want to partner with me to make an out-of-this-world, healthy, tasty cookbook, please contact my agent Kristin Nelson—she'll be happy to talk to you.

And now I am getting WAY off track. My point is that I spent several months during the summer watching documentary after documentary on food production and farming, and their effects on our environment. If you care about what goes into your body and how it gets there, I would HIGHLY suggest checking out a few of those. I need to know that several different sources confirm the same things before I will incorporate changes that will affect my family.

One documentary I watched really impacted me about our consumption of beef and the impact the beef industry has on the environment. One of our children was also similarly impacted, and she asked me if we could simply switch out some of the beef we were eating to turkey or chicken. It didn't seem like that big of a thing to do, so we bought almost all ground turkey to substitute for the beef.

Two important things I want to share that came from this simple experiment. First, our grocery bills went way down! I feed 10 people three times each day and that adds up REAL quick, so I'm as frugal as I can be with my grocery shopping. I was so happy to see that our costs went down considerably just switching from beef to turkey and chicken.

Initially, I thought *maybe* some of the recipes would work with this change, and I didn't know what my kids would have to say about the changes. Which leads me to the second point: My kids prefer the ground turkey to the beef. They *rave* about my turkey meat sauce, meatballs, and meatloaf. Even my husband agreed this was a good change.

Now, I'm not suggesting you need to totally eliminate red meat, but cutting back improves health, saves money, and helps the environment, which is only going to make Mama happier, right? I was thrilled. Later, in the recipe section, I'll share some of our favorite switch-ups using ground turkey and chicken.

Depending on your family members, you might want to try and hide the change, or talk to them about why you've decided to switch things up. I have the sort of kids who love to be involved in what I'm learning, and they like to discuss it with us. Our three older kids talk about these things with their friends and teachers, too. At this point they might even know more than I do! You know your kids best, so make the decision that seems right for your family. You might even mix some beef and some ground turkey at first just to be super sneaky! I am totally okay with sneaking things in on my little boys and my husband. I think I was putting kale, spinach, and okra into their smoothies for months before they finally caught me. Once they realized they liked it and were used to it, they couldn't even complain . . . much.

I also had another huge *aha!* moment during this time. Each night we have a "family question" during dinner and each person at the table has to answer. Sometimes it's a really thoughtful question like, "What was the hardest part of your day?" Other times, it is something silly like "if you could be any animal, which animal would you be?" Well, one night I asked the kids what their favorite meat was because, honestly, I just couldn't think of another question. Do you know what every single one of my kids said except for one? *FISH*?! WTF! I had no clue my kids even *liked* fish that much. Even the two little boys! Who were these kids and where did they come from?

It just continually blows my mind how their eating habits have changed. So now I'm trying to do one meal with fish each week. I can often find great sales on frozen wild salmon, which isn't cheap, but a bag for $5 or $6 really isn't bad either when you consider how healthy it is for them. We really love adding the FLAVORGOD seasonings to fish too—the ranch and cheese flavors are a huge hit with the kids.

I often get comments about how expensive these flavorings are, but I buy them when they're on sale, and they last quite a while. When you can sprinkle chicken, salad, or fish with a seasoning that the kids gobble up, it becomes worth it. Give it a try!

One thing I've seen over and over again is how little protein most people consume. I think this is often why stalls or slow-downs happen. If we keep reducing the amount of food we are consuming, and push harder with exercise, we create a starvation mode in the body. Then we get frustrated, and it becomes a crazy, vicious cycle. *Please*, don't underestimate how important protein is to your health!

If you aren't sure what your protein macronutrient goals are, there are several free websites that will give you a good range. Here's a great one: healthyeater.com/flexible-dieting-calculator. I try to include protein in each and every meal and snack. You can easily add protein powder to almost anything if you need a quick fix. Below is a list of some of my favorite protein choices.

I recommend:

- Greek Yogurt
- Cottage Cheese
- Eggs
- Whey Isolate Protein (Jay Robb brand is the best, in my opinion)
- Chicken Breast (Boneless Skinless)
- Turkey Breast
- Tuna
- Salmon
- Tilapia
- Beans
- Lentils
- Peanut or Almond butter
- Nuts
- Quinoa

Jay Robb whey isolate protein powder is our family go-to. It has the best, most ideal ingredients available, and you can even order it from Amazon at a really great discount and have it delivered right to your door! You can't beat that! We add it to shakes, smoothies, pudding, yogurt, pancakes, and waffles. One of my favorite breakfasts is egg white French toast with cottage cheese and blueberries on top. I always add vanilla-flavored Jay Robb to my cottage cheese and then sprinkle some cinnamon on top to give it sweetness and flavor. This breakfast is *packed* with fiber, protein, and healthy carbs, and it provides a great boost of energy. Particularly if I'm working out, running, or doing errands with the family, this breakfast will give me all I need to fuel my body at the start of the day.

Don't skimp on your breakfast. I know it's a cliché, but it's *so* important, and protein should always be the focus. I probably sound like a broken record about this, but it really is true. You can't drive a car without gas, but we often push ourselves to do the things we want our body to do without the proper fuel and nutrition. Then, we wonder why we are tired, sick, or physically fatigued. I firmly believe we often fuel our vehicles and homes better then we fuel our bodies. We would never throw junk into the engine of our car, but we routinely and mindlessly throw garbage into our bodies without a second thought.

Be mindful. Fill your body with care and consideration, because you are *worth* it, friend. Your body is the only one you're going to get. We can roll up to the dealership and easily get an upgrade on our cars, but we don't have that luxury with our bodies. We need to relearn self-care and it begins with fueling the beautiful machines we live in with the best possible food.

Pick your protein, healthy carbs, and fats wisely. They aren't created equally, and the results will all depend on your choices. I want you to have a fierce, strong, healthy machine. You deserve it! Remember your body WANTS to heal, it *wants* to be healthy and strong.

I know it's especially hard for us mamas to make choices that prioritize ourselves—we're usually at the very bottom of the list. I hear from so many women that it's going to be so difficult to rearrange a budget and make time for health and nutritional choices. But let me be clear: if *you* aren't in good health, everything in the life of your family will suffer. Your food choices are important. Your exercise and movement time are important. Not only for physical wellbeing, but for mental health too! So please, Mama, make good choices, make time so you can be the best you for your family for a very long time. Trust me when I say taking care of yourself will be contagious. Once you start, your body will crave more and more healthy changes. Just ask several of my beta readers, many of whom went on to quit smoking after they started eating clean.

Once you get on the road to health and wellness, you'll want more and more of it for yourself and your family.

Chapter 14

THE TRUE IMPORTANCE OF A CLEAN, WHOLE FOOD, CHEMICAL-FREE DIET

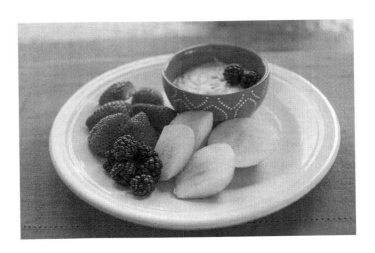

As MY FAMILY CONTINUES ON THIS JOURNEY, AND THE MORE I've studied, the more shocked and outraged I've become at the food industry. They've built their industry around our poor choices and capitalized that into a whole host of "food-like substances" that are so different from the truly nourishing and healing foods our grandparents made and enjoyed.

Now we spend our days being constantly hungry and unsatisfied.

We crave unhealthy things because our food is being genetically modified, and that compels us to eat more of what is killing us. As bold a statement that might be, it's that truth.

We weren't created to crave Pop Tarts, sugary cereals, cakes, and cookies. These products are intentionally designed to trigger our brains in such a way that we literally can't help ourselves. These products are everywhere we look; 80% of the grocery store shelves are filled with them. How are we supposed to make a change to our health when this is ingrained into our American lifestyle?

It really can be difficult to make changes, but not impossible. My best advice is to make using clean, non-GMO food a top priority. Food, how we get it, what it is, and what's in it really isn't something we think about. As our health continues to decline, I think it's absolutely imperative that we push other things a bit lower on our priority list and put our food choices at the top. Not only should we know what we're putting inside of us, but we really need to look at how it got there, too.

In researching whole foods, I couldn't believe the list of products grown by genetic modification. To be totally honest, I didn't even understand why this was happening. When it comes down to it, this isn't about food color or seedless varieties, as I'd once assumed; this is all about money. Crops are being modified via gene splicing to make them virtually un-killable by pesticide, so the food companies can make bigger profits. It's expensive to farm organic, and cheap to spray mass-produced pesticide poisons on the crops. This genetic modification is being done by the biggest chemical corporations who, it's important to note, also make many of the drugs used to treat our countless illnesses, most of which have only *cropped up* recently. I'll let you draw your own conclusions here.

The scariest issue is that, to date, there have been ZERO long-term independent studies on the safety of GMOs to humans. None. Nada. Not one. Also alarming is that GMO (genetically modified organism) seeds often infest the fields of farmers who aren't even using them, which causes GMOs to spread like wildfire. Researching this has scared the shit out of me. Will our grandchildren live to see and taste natural, God-made fruits and vegetables? As childhood cancers begin to rise alongside the inclusion of more and more chemicals and GMOs in our foods, I'm scared about the nutritional choices of future generations. *Please*, be informed about what you're feeding our children. Don't trust our food industry to put your health, or the health of your family, as a priority. This lies in our hands.

Jack and I have personally made changes about how our money and time is spent. We try to make the health of our family our top priority, and I urge you to do the same.

When you go grocery shopping, I highly recommend finding a local farmers co-op or market in your area, or shopping at organic, non-GMO grocery stores like Whole Foods, Spouts, Aldi, or Trader Joes. The other important thing is to read the labels. Below are some tips you might want to keep in mind when you go to buy your groceries:

Shopping Tips

The most important foods to buy that are organic/non-GMO:

- dairy
- meat
- corn
- zucchini
- yellow squash
- leafy greens
- berries

- bell peppers
- apples
- celery
- cherry tomatoes
- cucumbers
- potatoes
- grapes
- hot peppers
- peaches
- eggs
- tea and coffee
- herbs and spices
- chocolate

Non-GMO crops currently being developed as GMO:
- soy
- corn
- cotton
- canola
- sugar beets
- zucchini
- yellow squash papaya
- alfalfa

Foods that could possibly contain GMO ingredients:
- Aspartame
- Baking powder
- Canola oil
- Caramel color
- Cellulose

- Citric acid
- Cobalamin (Vitamin B12)
- Colorose
- Condensed milk
- Confectioners' sugar
- Corn flour
- Corn masa
- Cornmeal
- Corn oil
- Corn starch
- Corn sugar
- Cottonseed oil
- Cyclodextrin
- Dextrin
- Dextrose
- Diacetyl
- Diglyceride
- Equal
- Erythritol
- Food starch
- Fructose
- Glucose
- Glutamate
- Glutamic acid
- Glycerides
- Glycerin
- Glycerol
- Glycerol monooleate
- Glycine
- Hemicellulose

- High-fructose corn syrup
- Hydrogenated starch
- Hydrolyzed vegetable protein
- Inositol
- Inverse syrup
- Inversol
- Invert sugar
- Isoflavones
- Lactic acid
- Lecithin
- Leucine
- Lysine
- Maltitol
- Malt
- Malt extract
- Maltodextrin
- Maltose
- Malt syrup
- Mannitol
- Methylcellulose
- Milk powder
- Milo starch
- Modified food starch
- Mono and diglycerides
- MSG
- NutraSweet
- Oleic acid
- Phenylalanine
- Phytic acid
- Protein isolate

- Shoyu
- Sorbitol
- Soy flour
- Soy isolates
- Soy lecithin
- Soy milk
- Soy oil
- Soy protein
- Soy protein isolate
- Soy sauce
- Starch
- Stearic acid
- Sugar (all kinds except cane)
- Tamari
- Tempeh
- Teriyaki marinade
- Textured vegetable protein
- Threonine
- Tocopherols
- Tofu
- Trehalose
- Triglyceride
- Vegetable fat
- Vegetable oil
- Vitamin B12
- Vitamin E
- Whey
- Whey powder
- Xanthan gum

NOTE: that some of these things even my computer program didn't recognize!

But back to my chapter on ingredient reading from the first book, if you, your mama, and your computer don't know what it is, don't put it in your body! Be informed and try to avoid these foods as much as possible, unless you know they are non-GMO as shown by the butterfly label: www.nongmoproject.org

You can even download the non-GMO shopping guide app to scan products for content information. Also, The Food Babe, Vani Hari, consistently updates lists of these ingredients. And remember to check your meats. Animals are often fed GMO grains, which then enter us from the meats and dairy we eat.

If you can't eat only non-GMO and organic, just try and do the best you can. I believe all reduction in exposure to these chemicals will help us. Please also keep an eye on all the oils added to things, especially at your favorite restaurants! Our family tries to stick to the three safest oils: coconut, olive, and avocado.

THE SICKENING 15—a list of things to try to avoid in your food
- GROWTH HORMONES IN MEAT
- ANTIBIOTICS
- PESTICIDES
- REFINED AND ENRICHED FLOUR
- BISPHENOL (BPA)
- HIGH-FRUCTOSE CORN SYRUP (HFCS)
- ARTIFICIAL SWEETENERS
- PRESERVATIVES
- TRANS FATS
- ARTIFICIAL AND NATURAL FLAVORS

- FOOD DYES
- DOUGH CONDITIONERS
- CARRAGEENAN
- MONOSODIUM GLUTAMATE (MSG)
- HEAVY METALS & NEUROTOXINS

PRO TIP: Yes, I know this might be overwhelming; I often feel the same way. My advice is to take an entire weekend to really investigate your local markets. Again, a farmers co-op or market will usually have lots of healthy produce options for you. Ask questions about their farming practices and if they are organic—I've found most farmers like to talk about this.

Once you know which products are best and what your family likes, it will take far less time to shop. I actually only hit the very outside rim of my local big box store, and it takes about half the time it once did for me to shop. It will get easier!

I also order many of our pantry items as subscribe-and-save items at Amazon. These things automatically ship in the frequency best for you; we usually do every other month at a 15% discount. You just can't beat that, especially when it comes right to your door. Make sure you consider that option, especially if you can't find something locally. The truth is the cleaner you eat, the better you will feel and the healthier and stronger you and your family will be.

Chapter 15

YOUR HAPPY WEIGHT VS YOUR GOAL WEIGHT

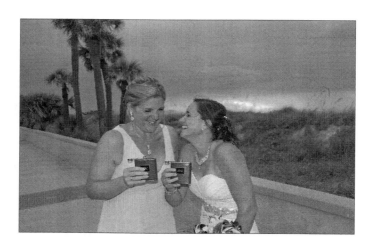

"To change the world/It starts with one step/However small/
First step is hardest of all."
—Dave Mathews Band

I ACTUALLY HATE THE TERM "GOAL WEIGHT." PROBABLY BECAUSE in my head, as a child, I knew I had about as much chance of achieving my "goal" weight as I had of flying. That had been an actual joke, a cruel joke. Even when I would basically starve myself as a child, the scale would go in the wrong direction. I faithfully ate my chemical-filled Weight Watchers meals and treats and yet, week after week, I just put on more and more weight. I believed I would never be able to meet any weight loss goals set by my doctor, nutritionist, or grandmother. My inability to meet their goals was a constant reminder of how bad I was, of how much of a failure I would always be. As sad as that might sound, it was exactly how I felt. So, I just filed away the idea of achieving a goal weight—it remained in the same category as my dream to be a rock star, or ride a unicycle, or travel to Australia.

When this health and wellness journey got me to my first mile-stone—losing 100 pounds—my doctor asked me if I had a goal in mind. Even though a goal had crossed my mind a few times, I really didn't have a specific number. At best, I had a large range of num-bers, and when I passed that goal I really had to ask myself what number would make me feel as if I had ended my journey.

But would it ever end? Would I ever really feel happy, satisfied, and comfortable in my body? All I had ever heard was the term "obese" over and over again my whole life. I knew I didn't want that term to be applied to me any longer. Size 12 sounded good. I didn't want to lose all of my curves; I wanted to look like a woman; I want-ed my legs to be strong and my butt to look full. Was there a number that would perfectly represent how I looked, *and* represent my new strength and health?

My quick answer to this question is . . . no.

In the same way there is no single word that can describe all of these things, neither can a hard and fast goal weight number. My journey is made up of many things: an amazing outfit, a particular moment, a special photo. In terms of weight, my journey is a collage of numbers.

As I mentioned before, even my two doctors couldn't agree on a good "goal range" for me. My primary care physician, who has a background in eating disorders and nutrition, had a range in her mind higher than my blood doctor had. Her reasoning had to do with muscle mass, and her worry was that if I got too small my body wouldn't be able to maintain my high muscle mass.

I also want to point out here that if you don't know your muscle mass and fat mass, you really should find out. Please don't rely on the outdated and largely irrelevant BMI (body mass index) as the best indicator of a physical goal for you. You can check out a calculator here: www.active.com/fitness/calculators/bodyfat. Even when my BMI said "obese" or "overweight," my fat percentage was in the acceptable range, because the BMI calculations don't take my muscle mass into consideration. Please don't believe one chart over the other, rather look at both and find a good in-between range in which you not only feel good, but also feel strong.

If you read *BIG GIRLS DO IT RUNNING*, you know I'm an advocate for not depriving myself. In fact, I think we should enjoy our treats, and I don't think we should waste time counting calories or putting food into tiny stupid boxes. I refuse to live my life that way.

So after lots of thought and prayer, I've decided that I won't set a goal weight number, just a goal *feeling*. When I get to the point where my body feels strong, healthy, and satisfied without any struggle, then I'll be where I'm supposed to be.

I don't think we need to pick an absolute number. What happens if you get to the place you always envisioned and you feel you still have work to do? What then? I've seen this happen several times. My mom only wanted to lose 10–15 pounds and then she kept losing and thought, gosh . . . maybe my body knows what it's doing, and I'll just keep going and trust it. Now, she's signed up for her first 10K and she's down over 20 lbs. She eats healthy, satisfying foods. She's happy, and she's off medications. Nanny Karri had almost the same experience. She just wanted to get under a certain number that she had never gotten under before; then she was below it. Then what? Well, she kept eating right and kept lifting her weights and running, and then she was five pounds under that number. Guess what? She's still going! She's gaining muscle and getting leaner, and she's faster than ever! I think her arms might even be more impressive than Jack's; please don't let him know I said that, but it's true!

Your happy weight might even be *higher* than you once thought. Maybe you started lifting weights and you realized, like me, that you LOVE it. Maybe you need to keep some of that weight and transfer it to muscle. That's great too! So what if it keeps you in the overweight BMI range if your fat percentage is 20%? That's great!

The real goal is all about how you *feel*. Can you run with your kids? Can you buy clothes at almost any store? Can you jump? Do you look in the mirror and smile back at what you see? Do you feel good when you have to weigh in for your doctor? Are you off those medications you've been on for years? These are the golden goals! They are what makes it all worth it, Mama!

Please don't let your happiness depend on some chart or number. And *please*, don't let some doctor let you believe that one old, outdated set of information is the only way to get a full and true picture of your health. If I have one prayer for each of you who are on this journey with me it's that you find your happy weight, that you find your strength, that you wear it boldly and proudly. Don't let anyone put Baby in the corner. This is Baby's turn to dance and have the time of her life. Yes, that was a dorky 80s movie reference.

I think we spend too much time feeling bad about ourselves, criticizing ourselves, and wanting what we don't have. I think it's time to stop letting these ridiculous standards and images hold us back. So often I see fitness posts about fitting into an outfit, or losing X amount of weight. Do we really need that to be the end point? Does that really define us? In our culture, these are the things that can really compromise our self-esteem.

I suggest to you that our health and our ability to live without the chains of food addiction, obsession, pain, and suffering is really where our dreams should be. I believe each of us has been created to be happy, satisfied, and nourished. Sadly, a lifetime of "food-like products" has caused our bodies to shut down and not work the way they should.

This isn't your fault.

Let me say it again: THIS IS NOT YOUR FAULT!

You aren't lazy, you don't have an issue with willpower—you've been *poisoned*. Once you've finally cleansed your body and are on the road to getting it healed, give it grace and give it time. Remember, this isn't a sprint, it's a marathon. Yes, there will be some ups and downs, you will get discouraged, you will get frustrated, but you'll also find great joy and better health. Hold on, and try to stick with me. Find your happy. Look for those daily moments where you see yourself in a positive way. Be proud of your continued better choices. Find a place where your body feels healthy, strong, and proud, and hold on tight!

I'm proud of you, so *you* be proud of you, too.

Chapter 16

HORMONES, CHOCOLATE, WINE, SUPPLEMENTS, AND OTHER THINGS THAT JUST POPPED INTO MY HEAD

BEING A WOMAN IS AMAZING, BUT SOMETIMES IT REALLY SUCKS. I can't tell you how many times I'm downright green with jealousy when my husband's body changes faster than mine, or that he doesn't have to contend with the five pound weight gain in the middle of the month, or that he doesn't have crazy carb and chocolate cravings, or pimples, or hot flashes. It just isn't fair!

Every month is an up and down battle between me and my hormones. My mom started "the change" when she hit 40 and, since I'm am overachiever, I'm pretty sure I'm riding the red bridge over there right now at age 37.

My mid-month weight gain and bloating, with the carb and chocolate cravings two weeks later, is enough to drive me insane. I probably won't ever have peace with this. It will always suck, but the good news is that the longer I've been on this journey and the cleaner and healthier I eat, the better my body seems to be with my monthly cycle. I often had horrible, painful periods that would last a full week, which would make my nutritional issues worse and, in turn, would necessitate iron infusions just to keep me from feeling horrible. I would become weak, lightheaded, and tired. It wasn't fun. As I continued to eat better, however, I found my periods only lasted three to four days, five at most. This was a wonderful side effect of my better food choices.

Most months I still have the carb and chocolate cravings, but instead of lasting for days, it's usually a few hours at night. I deal with it by snacking on some dark chocolate and healthy popcorn. This happens almost every month like clockwork—it never fails. The funny part is Jack knows right when this happens, and he always has the necessary supplies ready for me.

I've learned to embrace this, now. There are going to be weeks during the month when my weight will go up because of hormones, and it's okay . . . it'll drop back down. There are going to be days when I need chocolate . . . BADLY. There are going to be days when I'll need an extra glass of wine, also totally okay. Please don't let those weeks, days, or hours be an excuse to give up—in fact, those can be days to celebrate.

Here's my best advice on when this happens: **HAVE A SAFTEY NET**! If you don't have healthy safety net foods in your house, or close by, it's easy to cave and eat something that you'll feel bad about later, causing a guilt spiral. I've seen this over and over again in my group. Listen to me, ladies: this is normal and 100% OKAY! I am done fighting my body. I am going to listen to the cues it gives me and embrace how it works. So if I'm a bit bloated or crabby I'm still going to put on my BIG GIRL exercise pants and work my body and fuel it well.

Another important thing I've learned this year is that I've been suffering—probably for a very long time—from severe adrenal fatigue. My doctor is actually the one who told me she wanted me to try an adrenal support supplement after I told her I was having more difficulty managing stress than usual.

I've said it before and I'll say it again: I think women today are just at higher levels of stress than ever before in the history of womanhood. Heck, life is exhausting, right? The same signals our body would have triggered if a dangerous animal was chasing us are now being triggered all day long. We're constantly in survival mode. We're depressed, stressed, and always at the end of our rope, and that isn't a stress our bodies were designed to sustain long-term.

I've usually been pretty good at dealing with stress—I manage motherhood, work, and marriage. Yes, sometimes I have bad days, but I'd never felt like my brain was shutting down when an especially stressful situation arose. In fact, I was at the point that I worried something else was going on. Was it just anxiety? A deeper level of anxiety?

The first day I took my adrenal support pills, I felt different. My brain was clearer, I slept better, I had better focus. I read a review on the herbal Gaia supplement I take that said if they ever won the lottery they would buy these for every single person they know, and I honestly have to say I can understand that. Now, I'm certainly not saying that EVERYONE in the world has adrenal fatigue, but I would guess many of you reading this right now might have it to some degree.

If you google adrenal fatigue you're going to get all sorts of contradictory information about it, but what my research has revealed is this: if you're dealing with lack of energy, anxiety, sudden and strong food cravings, allergies, difficulty in performing daily tasks, difficulty focusing, depression, difficulty sleeping, intense sensitivity to cold and/or dizziness then this might be something to talk to your doctor about. (BTW, this is the *short* list, people; there are countless other issues linked to adrenal fatigue.)

When I looked into it, I decided trying the support supplement was worth a shot, just to see if any of these conditions improved. I have to say that it has been a huge relief to be able to manage these symptoms by taking the supplement. I take them daily in addition to my ACV, multivitamin, and probiotic. They've been a literal miracle for my mind. We are still doing collagen and MCT oil too; collagen usually goes into our post-workout shakes as we've found that is the easiest way to get it in; MCT is great in our morning coffee.

Figure out what works best for you. I know some people have told me they mix the collagen, MCT, stevia drops, and cream all together in their morning coffee, and others put the MCT or collagen in soup or tea. Any way you can get those in will be good for your body. I can't tell you how much my hair, nails, and skin has changed because of those small doses of collagen in my shakes and smoothies. It's a big wow. Don't believe me? Just try it for 30 days and see what you think. I get comments almost daily about how young I look, and I truly believe the fountain of youth comes from what we are putting *in* our bodies.

Speaking of the fountain of youth, I want to update you about my skin care. I am still using the vitamin C serum faithfully—I really feel this has helped with the overall condition of my skin. We've also really tried to find products for bath and body that are as clean and organic as possible. When I first looked at those products during a trip to Whole Foods, I was shocked by the prices. Now you can find good, high quality, organic products at much better prices, especially on Amazon if you do the subscribe-and-save option; 15% off and sent right to my door whenever I want it. Sounds like a great idea to me! The Art Naturals and Beauty by Earth products are awesome, and Puracy has been a great bath care line for my kids. There are so many great, reasonably priced natural and organic products out there now. If you can get those for the same cost as the chemical-filled brands, why not buy the natural and better-for-your- body-ones? Your skin is your body's largest organ, so don't neglect it! If you wouldn't put it on your skin, don't put it in your mouth, and if you wouldn't put it in your mouth, don't put it on your skin.

Chapter 17

VEGGIES, PALATE CHANGES, AND THE WILDER WAY

by Jack Wilder

I HATE VEGETABLES. IF YOU'VE READ *BIG GIRLS DO IT RUNNING*, you know this already. I've hated vegetables my whole life. Just ask my mother, she'll tell you. In fact, I can think of a story from my childhood that may illustrate how far back and how deeply ingrained my dislike of veggies really goes.

When I was a kid, my parents had a hard and inviolable rule: you don't get down from the table until your plate is cleared, ESPECIALLY OF VEGETABLES. I swear they made that rule up just to troll me. I mean, maybe not, they may have just wanted me to be healthy and eat my veggies, since everyone knows veggies are good for you. But as a stubborn three-year-old? It was a rule designed to torture me. I'd eat my chicken, I'd eat spaghetti, I'd eat meatloaf, I'd eat potatoes and rice and bread and corn and whatever else, but veggies? NOPE.

The story goes like this, as I remember it, with a few details provided by my mom:

Family dinner—my mom and dad, my older sister, and me. I don't remember what the main dish was, probably Mom's special chicken paprika with a baked potato . . . and lima beans—my arch nemesis. I ate the chicken and I ate the potatoes, but I just couldn't stomach the lima beans. To me they tasted like an old gym shoe mixed with Elmer's glue and moldy Satan hork. Nope, nope, nope. So I delayed. I tried all my tactics—whining, crying, refusing, arguing, pushing them around the plate so it looked like there were fewer beans . . . but to no avail.

"You're not leaving the table until you finish ALL of the lima beans, Jack," my dad insisted.

But . . . I wanted to *play*. As it was, I'd been at the table for something like an hour and a half already, because I was the slowest eater in the family. Mom and Dad were done, and my older sister had eaten her food and was in her room playing already—I spent my childhood absolutely convinced my sister used to sneak her veggies onto my plate . . . and years later she actually admitted that she DID do that, now and then. So yeah, just little three-year-old Jack by himself at the big old table with a plate full of veggies, my toys calling my name . . .

And a set of parents who insisted I couldn't leave the table until it was clear of all veggies. I'm not usually a very literal person, but at that point, I was at my wit's end. So I took their words literally: I shoved all the Satan beans—I mean lima beans—into my mouth, chewed them enough so my cheeks weren't bulging, and then got down from the table and started playing.

Over an hour later, my mom asked me a question, and I couldn't respond, since I had a mouthful of lima beans. My mom realized what I'd done, and how long I'd been on the floor playing with a mouthful of partially masticated lima beans, and finally realized how committed I was to the cause of not eating lima beans. She let me spit them out and never forced me to eat lima beans again, although the war to get Jack to eat his veggies waged on for the rest of my life.

I haven't touched a lima bean since, and will not until my dying day.

When we were first married, Jasinda was unaware of my hatred of that food. She once made a frozen veggie medley for dinner and it contained lima beans. I had an epic tantrum, which led to me telling her this same story, and announcing that there was no force on earth that could make me eat lima beans.

That hasn't changed. That will *never* change. I call it a traumatic incident involving lima beans, kind of like lima bean PTSD. The rest of my childhood, as I said, was punctuated with daily fights to get me to eat broccoli, green beans, peas, etc., with my parents usually winning. When I grew up and moved out, I stopped eating veggies entirely, at least partially because I ate like a bachelor: e.g. fast food, canned chili and soup, pizza, and all that garbage. Then I married Jasinda, and we had kids, and I had to start eating like an adult, meaning real meals with real food . . . and VEGETABLES.

"You have to set an example for the kids, Jack," my wife would tell me, usually accompanied by her distinctly Jasinda eye-roll. "So try to eat at least SOME veggies and not make a big deal about it, so the kids will eat them."

Joke's on me, though, because even before we started the Wilder Way, our older kids all discovered that they *loved* broccoli and were willingly to eat most other veggies. Our oldest daughter *LOVES* Brussels sprouts, which is still utterly baffling to me.

It was my younger boys I had to set an example for, so I had to eat my veggies and act like it wasn't torture all over again.

"You'll learn to like veggies when you're older, Jack," my parents used to tell me. Yet, whenever the subject of vegetables came up as an adult, I'd insist that I was pretty sure I *was* older now, and I *still* didn't like them.

Well . . . enter the #WilderWay.

As you're no doubt familiar, we started small. We cut out sugar at breakfast, and then at lunch, and then at dinner, and then we cut out all sodas and sugary drinks. And then we eliminated all processed foods and pre-packaged carbs. At the same time, we started adding in new foods, most of which I'd always insisted I didn't like.

And, at first, I didn't.

Sweet potatoes were one of the first things we started adding. I had a hard time with that. I didn't like the texture, and really hated the flavor, with the rare exception of sweet potato French fries, if they were cooked extra crispy. Then Jasinda and Nanny Karri started making these sweet potato sliders, which are baked slices of sweet potato, chunks of chicken breast, chicken bacon, and some kind of delicious ranch or Greek yogurt sauce with lots of spices and FLAVORGOD seasoning . . . I think the recipe is in the back. I wasn't sure about them at first, but I ate them. The next time, I was like, eh, I guess they're okay. And now, a few months later, I look forward to them . . . especially if my sliders have the sweet potatoes baked extra crispy.

It's the same story with avocado and guacamole and broccoli. I never really hated broccoli, I just didn't care for it. And then my wife started making broccoli with lots of spicy stuff on it, cayenne and chili powder and Everything Spicy FLAVORGOD, and lots of garlic . . . and I'd find myself adding more to my plate. It wasn't immediate—it took a few months of detox, and gradual palate change, and just plain old eating it. I knew it was good for me and I had to set an example for my kids. And I did learn to like broccoli.

Avocado was a surprise to me. I'd tried guac a few times and was just . . . meh. Don't hate it, but don't love it, won't eat it. Then we started adding avocado to things like sliders and sandwiches and burrito bowls and tacos and breakfast burritos, and I realized . . . holy heck, I *like* it. So we bought a container of organic, non-GMO, spicy guacamole, and I ate it with the Red Hot Blues corn chips . . . and I *loved* it. You could've knocked me over with a feather when I realized this. I'd just assumed I still didn't like it, and then suddenly I did. It was like magic.

Green beans? Meh. Steam them and serve them plain? Ugh-UH!—as our little boys say. Add spices and some flavor and seasoning? Yum!

My point is this: give yourself time. Give your kids time. Give your husband time. You've been eating the same kinds of foods your whole life. As humans, we fall into ruts, and we sink into familiar patterns. At some point we just decide we don't like salad, or veggies, or sweet potatoes, so we eat other stuff and just keep avoiding those things out of habit. We pick up a bag of chips because it's quick and easy and tasty. We stop for McDonalds because it's on the way home and it's already 5:30, and by the time we get home and put together a meal and eat it'll be 6:45. The kids should start getting ready for bed at 7:30. I'm *tired,* and cooking sounds like a *horrible* idea. Or heck, it's Saturday, let's just order a pizza. Quick, easy, tasty.

It's habit. It's convenient. I did it my whole life, and for most of my kids' lives.

And then we forced ourselves to examine our eating habits, the reasoning behind them, and—even more difficult—we examined the consequences of those habits: all this junk food is quick and easy, but it's killing us. It's making us fat and lazy and weak and slow—I'm talking about myself, here. That was me, and I didn't even realize it. But then my wife had her *aha!* moment and introduced the Wilder Way to our family and, by degrees and in increments, I discovered new energy, new strength, new motivation . . . and a new palate for food.

I wouldn't eat fast food now if *you* paid *me*. I wouldn't eat regular pizza, or donuts, or chips, or candy, or the most decadent chocolate-y dessert you could find. I wouldn't. I *couldn't*. The very thought literally turns my stomach. This didn't happen immediately, and it wasn't even necessarily fast, but the change happened. The same is true for our younger kids. For them, it's still happening. We sometimes still have to cajole them into eating their veggies, but they do eat them, and every time the fight is shorter, and I know eventually they'll stop fighting it altogether, because their tastes will have changed.

Consistency is the key to this. We always offer our kids healthy snacks, now. Before the Wilder Way, our kids ate the hot lunch at school, which was whatever was on offer. Our kids go to a small local elementary which actually provides healthier-than-usual school lunches, but as we embarked on this nutrition journey, we realized that for our kids to truly have the healthiest lunch possible, we'd need to send them with lunches from home. We make them cold cut wraps, PB+J sandwiches on sprouted bread, soups they can heat in the microwave at school, all with sides of blue corn chips, healthy popcorn, sliced fruit . . . and veggies.

At first, the veggies came back uneaten, especially in the younger boys' lunches. And then, over time, the carrots, cucumbers, celery, red, green, and yellow peppers, and even the sugar snap peas and raw broccoli would get eaten, especially if they had something yummy to dip them in, like some Greek yogurt with some ranch FLAVORGOD mixed in. Then, when they get home, we usually have a spread of veggies and dip on the counter, and they'll munch on those too as they settle in from school . . . and so do I, actually.

Another change we made was to offer a salad bar at every dinner.

And I do mean every single dinner. There's a big bowl of spring mix or power greens, and several smaller bowls filled with diced carrots, cucumbers, tomatoes, celery, and peppers, with several different kinds of dressing on option. This is yet another way to allow the kids to make their own choices about how they want to eat veggies. Now, everyone eats a salad at least once a day.

There are always fresh veggies in our house, and they're quickly becoming a staple snack, to replace other, less healthy alternatives. But it wasn't always this way; it consistently took offering these foods to our kids—and to me, if I'm being honest—for the habit of eating fresh veggies to take hold. And now, like everything else on the Wilder Way, it's just become a way of life.

And that, at its core, is what makes this plan my wife has created so special: it's not a diet, it's not a fad, it's not a gimmick, there are no secrets or tricks or sneaky money-grab products or plans to buy separately; it's just simple nutritious eating as a lifestyle.

Simple doesn't mean easy, obviously, as there is a learning curve, but the farther down this path you go, the easier it becomes, because your tastes just . . . change. Especially when you reach the point where the unhealthy poison food-like products just aren't an option anymore . . . that's when you really start moving and learning and making this a lifestyle. We modify, we tweak, we offer healthy alternatives at every meal, every day, consistently, making it easy for our kids—and ourselves—to eat the healthiest possible foods.

Humans are incredibly adaptable; this is a well-known fact. Put a group of people in the Antarctic, and after a few months they'll be going outside in the sub-zero temperatures in shirt-sleeves. I've seen it, and I've experienced it myself. I live in northern Michigan where the temperatures routinely dip well below zero in the winter. During the first few weeks of winter I'm always cold, but I intentionally allow myself to be exposed to the cold on a regular basis. By January or February, I can go outside in 10- or 20-degree weather in a T-shirt and light coat unless I'm going to be outside for long periods. Same with heat, or pain, or pleasure. Anything we're exposed to regularly, we adapt to, become accustomed to.

This applies to food, as well. At first, veggies are icky; that's a habit, that's a preconceived notion, an acquired taste. But if we season them—make them spicy, or garlicky, or whatever—and eat them regularly, we'll learn to tolerate them, and eventually learn to like them. The difference is, the seasons change, summer comes, and we're none the worse for wear from the temperature. With food, however, the price of subjecting our bodies to garbage "food-like products" such as fast food, pizza, and convenient store junk like Pop Tarts or candy or donuts or whatever, is very serious. Our bodies are being poisoned, our metabolisms are slowing down, our arteries are becoming clogged, our brain functions are impaired, and our immune systems are being weakened which, in turn, makes us susceptible to all sorts of diseases and illnesses . . .

Or, we can train our bodies and palates to enjoy healthy, nutritious food, and we'll detox from the junk and, in time, our bodies—these adaptable, incredible, self-healing machines—will purge the toxins, and repair the damage, and our metabolisms will jumpstart, and suddenly we will feel like we *can* run three miles or six miles, or do 80 pushups, or do 25 pull-ups with a 25 lb weight attached to us, or carry our 170 lb younger brother on our back, up the stairs, at a jog. These changes will not be immediate; it will take time, it will take training, and it will take consistency.

It all starts small. Just *try* it. Stick with it. Keep trying. Always try new things, and don't just try them once, try them a dozen times and in different ways. Give your body and your taste buds time to adjust, especially if you're just starting out on the Wilder Way.

I still won't eat lima beans; that's a hard and fast limit for me. Bring on just about anything else, though, and I will probably learn to like it. Just give me time.

Chapter 18

WILDER KIDS—STRONG AND HEALTHY

I AM GOING TO TALK TO YOU LIKE WE'RE BEST FRIENDS SITTING AT lunch and chatting over a nice glass of red wine. I have so much to say about the current state of the health of our children in this country. I am not going to hold anything back because I don't think we have time for pulling punches or political correctness. I believe that the future for our kids is dependent on the choices we make today.

I want to explain to you the difference in my kids from before we started taking our nutrition seriously and today. The best words I can use are night and day—not only are my kids now leaps and bounds healthier than they were, but they are stronger as well. They see themselves as athletic. They run! They run FAST! My two oldest sons have received medals in races that were even difficult for my husband to finish. They are finally feeling like their bodies can do amazing things. They WANT to try new things with us in the gym. As two parents who really weren't athletic at all, it's so cool to see.

Here's a shocking statistic for you: data published in the Journal of American Medical Association showed that 31.8 percent of youths ages 2–19 are overweight and, even worse, 16.9 percent are classified as obese—and these numbers continues to grow. Studies also suggest that overweight and obese children become overweight adults who suffer serious health problems and diseases. Even more shocking is that this generation could even have a lower life expectancy than their parents. Looking at the current studies and projections on health in America, I believe the present situation is grave. My heart aches for the kids who are currently struggling with obesity like I did. It brings me to tears just thinking about it.

So, what can we do? How can we teach our children about real nutrition and real food? How can we teach them to move their bodies and to get excited about exercise?

As I write this I'm on a school trip with my daughter, and the ages of the kids are between 10–18 years. Each morning we're offered a "healthy" continental breakfast at the hotel and the choices available include sugary cereal, fruit juice, bagels, sugar-filled yogurt, melon, and pineapple. There wasn't even a single apple in sight! After perusing the options, my daughter and I decide to stick to our protein bars.

What shocks me is that when I watch these kids eating, I estimate each child is consuming anywhere from 50–100 grams of sugar, *just at breakfast*, and some were probably getting over 100 grams! And most of these kids are totally unaware that eating four regular-sized candy bars would have the same effect on their bodies as what they are eating at the continental breakfast.

How can we teach our kids about health when we don't even give them healthy options?

Moms, I urge you to talk about nutrition with your kids. There's a lifetime of horrible health consequences on the horizon for our future generations if we don't make serious and immediate changes.

We might be close to producing a generation with a *lower* life expectancy than ours if things don't change, and only we can change it.

Please consider this: a breakfast muffin can contain 46 grams of sugar where a cupcake would have 34 grams; one serving of a popular breakfast yogurt has 15 grams of sugar, the same as a ½ cup of ice cream; the granola bar your kid takes to school for a "healthy" snack has as much added sugar as a full-sized candy bar; pancakes have as much sugar as a big slice of cheesecake, and a serving of granola cereal has more sugar than five Oreo cookies! These are examples from the typical American breakfast . . . and then we wonder why our kids need medications.

They have bad grades, they can't poop, and they're restless at night. Folks, this is because they're inflamed and sugar-high on a daily basis. I get emails DAILY from moms who have seen dramatic changes in their kids after getting them off sugar: their grades improve, they go off medications, and they hear from teachers that their kids are just different kids. This isn't surprising to me, because I saw this with my own children. I believe the effects of sugar on their developing bodies are vast and lasting. Just one such effect—the one most often talked about—is obesity, but there is a vast array of other effects equally as severe. Moms, if your child has a difficult time sleeping, suffers from allergies, bowel issues, skin issues, or has trouble concentrating, *PLEASE*, try to get them off sugar. If you can't do it completely then, at the very least, try to cut the added sugars from their diet as much as possible.

Below are some quick #WilderWay snacks that most kids enjoy:
- Oikos 000 yogurt. Kids love this. There is no added sugar, so it's a great choice.
- WASA or sprouted bread sandwiches

- Dreamfields or brown rice pasta
- Fair Life milk
- True Lemon and Lime—my kids all take these packets to school daily
- Zevia soda
- Mission or Joseph wrap pizza or pizza pockets
- Veggies and fruit dressed up with fancy shapes or dips
- Progresso Light chicken noodle soup (My kids love taking this to lunch with some Wasa crackers and Laughing Cow cheese)
- Halo Top ice cream
- Smoothies and Green Juice! These are a favorite of both of the Wilder girls. My youngest begs for her green juice by bringing us her cup and yelling, "juice!"

Just as I recommend for adults, I really think that removing sugar gradually is the way to go. Remember that they can also go through withdrawal and detox symptoms, so it might be tough at first, but the positive changes and results you will see are worth it. You can do it, Mama! I know your kids will thank you for it one day even if the cries and screams now say otherwise.

This doesn't need to happen overnight. You can start by just switching out a few things that contain the highest amounts of added sugar. That alone will have a huge impact on your child's health over time. And then, after a few months, switch out a few more things. I'll say it again and again—this isn't a sprint, it's a marathon. Rome wasn't built in a day and Jack Wilder didn't start eating veggies in a week. Give your kids time and keep offering healthier choices. They are worth it!

PRO TIP: Want to really enjoy your family dinner? Dim the lights and put some candles on the table. I'm amazed how much better my kids behave and how much better they eat when I light some candles to set the mood for dinner. It doesn't take much time or money, but this simple trick can make all the difference between dinner feeling like fast food, or a special meal for the kids.

Chapter 19

IF THE #WILDERWAY WORKS, WHY DO WE NEED THE 2.0?

WHEN I ANNOUNCED I WAS WORKING ON A 2.0 FOR MY program I immediately got questions from people asking why my program needed any changes if it already worked so well. To be totally honest, after a year and a half of carb cycling and wogging, I just wanted to mix things up and see what my body's response would be. I was so happily surprised with the changes I experienced that I thought it was important for me to share these things with you.

First, I *still* had issues with carbs and my hunger when I was working out harder. I've learned that carbs DO make me want to eat more frequently. I'm listening to my body and allowing myself to EAT MORE CARBS! Hallelujah!

Second, I really liked the idea of alternating carb days and fats days based on the intensity of my workouts. I liked the extra energy I got from the carbs on my harder workout days. Why not just use that day to fully enjoy my carbs and let them give me extra energy for lifting, rowing, pushing, and pulling? I also found I felt more satisfied, and my body felt better. Then, on the days I was focusing on fats I would do core work, or just a lighter workout . . . and gosh, that felt good, too!

Now, do I think everyone will have the same response to this alternating pattern? Probably not, but I think it's great to keep your body guessing while separating fuels. In my beta testing, we found that inches lost and shape toning really seemed to improve with these adjustments. Muscle built up more quickly, and we all just felt so much stronger.

A huge plus for these changes was that it made meal planning and grocery shopping so much easier, since we knew from week to week exactly how much of everything we needed. For us, it really simplified our food intake—typically, we would take all of our favorite meals for Black Plate days and for White Plate days and put them in a rotation. We also found that we didn't get sick of things as easily because when you're going a day or two without either fats or carbs you get excited about having them again.

The other strange thing is that we started trying new foods to replace or tweak things we usually enjoyed. For example, none of my family was ever really into sweet potatoes; maybe one or two of the kids would eat them. Once we began our revised White Plate days, I tried different ways to bring in those healthy carbs. Sweet potatoes sliders, sweet potato waffles, sweet potato pizza—these all became dishes my family asked for.

It was the same with avocados. Even six months ago, none of my family liked avocado, and most of my family would stick out a tongue if I even suggested guacamole. I needed to get more of those healthy fats in, so I started sneaking avocado into salads, wraps, and even shakes! Guess what? Now, my family is asking for avocado all the time.

I've also become more creative with plain yogurt and cottage cheese; I can't believe how many things I've adjusted for us just by using plain Greek yogurt. Yes, it does take a bit more time and prep, but it's been cheaper and it's so much healthier for us.

Try and become a bit adventurous yourselves. And, yes, I've got a few of our favorite 2.0 recipes for you later in this book, so don't worry. I just want to encourage you to try and tweak the things you like the most. Maybe you've always LOVED making zucchini bread—well, guess what? You still can! There's almost nothing you can't make healthier with a few modifications. If you need some ideas just get on Pinterest and put in "low carb, no sugar _____", and something will pop up to inspire you. Even Grandma's famous jelly cookies!

My favorite way to look for new recipes, or ways to modify recipes, is to go to Pinterest. I know people get hangry because I don't share more recipes but, honestly, most of my recipes are simple things, old family favorites that I modify, or things I find on Pinterest while browsing for ideas. You can do this, too. Even if you can't find something exactly like what you've made before, you should be able to find some ideas for something as tasty, or even better! I promise!

Now for the physical changes.

I am going to be totally and completely honest with you and say that adding strength training to my fitness regimen was just me trying to get more bang from my exercise time. Could I get the same sort of fat burning and strengthening workout in *less* time? Ladies, I have to be totally honest: I just don't have an hour or more to spend running or in the gym every day. I really wish I did, but I don't. Maybe once all of the kids are in school, or when I don't have a hundred animals, or when life isn't so busy and Jack and I are living a life of leisure. Who am I kidding? That's never going to happen for us. I wish it would, but we just have too much on our plates to devote a lot of time to working out.

And anyway, who *really* wants to spend that much time working out when there are so many other amazing things to do? So, I really wanted to try some high intensity options to see if I could get similar or even better results in less time. My goal was half an hour—30 minutes, or about 2% of your day. Come on, everyone can manage that, right? I also wanted to use minimal equipment.

I don't have time to even drive to the gym—and I'm not judging those who do, or those who *like* to go to the gym—I just know it doesn't work for me. I have a hard enough time getting to the grocery store to feed us all.

So, this new compact and challenging workout routine REALLY worked well for me. On White Plate days we typically go a bit longer with our workout—maybe up to 45 minutes—but for Black Plate days we really try and stick with a quick and dirty 30-minute workout, and we try to push as hard as we can in those 30 minutes.

Often I'll start with a one-mile sprint and then do some high intensity metcons to really get things burning. What's a metcon? A metcon is just METabolic CONditioning, a staple of crossfit training. You repeat the same two to three exercises in a series of rounds. Often we do as many rounds as we can in the last 5 or 6 of those 30 minutes. You'd be surprised how many squats, jumping jacks, push-ups, or burpees you can do in that time.

We also try to increase our speed and get more rounds into that time. The other awesome benefit of training this way was that we saw our running speeds improve as well as increased toning and fat burning. This also REALLY works well for the colder times of the year when a three-mile run just doesn't sound very appealing in the -20 degree temps we can get in northern Michigan.

I also like to mix up some of our workouts to include other fun things that we enjoy. Nanny Karri and I like to do power yoga on occasion, and I even did a tap workout with my daughter. By offering flexibility and options to your workout, you will remain excited and interested in challenging your body in different ways. There are so many things you can do to get your heart rate up and move your body.

Dr. K recently told me that most people are in poor health because they lose motivation and give up. Maybe many of them are just bored? Try to keep challenging yourself! Push yourself. Give yourself a reason to keep going and trying new things!

Our family has recently set some group running goals. We really want to do a Disney run, and my husband decided he wants to run a full Marathon. Please don't get me wrong, I'm not at all saying you have to run a marathon, but you can certainly try to increase your running distance or speed. Maybe you might want to try a new sport—one of the ladies in my Facebook group just joined an adult soccer team. How fun does that sound? I am sure you can find something that not only increase your strength and improves your health, but also brings more joy into your life, too.

Here are a few more of my exercise ideas that you might want to try:

- Aerobics
- Ballet or other dance classes
- Baseball
- Basketball
- Biking
- Bowling
- Boxing
- Canoeing
- Dancing
- Football

- Frisbee
- Golf
- Gymnastics
- Hiking
- Hockey
- Hopscotch
- Horseback Riding—one of my favorites
- Hula hooping
- Ice Skating
- Jogging
- Jump rope
- Laser tag
- Paddleboard
- Paintball
- Ping-Pong—my grandmother played until the day she died!
- Playing catch
- Rock climbing
- Rollerblading
- Rollerskating
- Running after your kids!
- Skateboarding
- Skiing
- Soccer
- Softball
- Swimming
- Tae Kwon Do or other martial arts
- Tennis
- Trampoline
- Treadmill
- Volleyball

- Walking
- Weightlifting

After all your activity, you should let yourself rest when you need rest. Give your body some time off. I've done that several times over the past two years, and I think it was really good for me. I'm not one to really "exercise" on vacation, so you won't see me in the hotel workout room. I work out way less when I'm on my period, and if I'm sick my workout will be just a bit of easy stretching or walking.

Working out and moving should IMPROVE how you feel and your quality of life, so if you're feeling yucky it's absolutely fine to give your body the time it needs to rest and heal. Just make sure you get right back into it as soon as you start feeling better. Nutrition should always be the focus no matter how you feel; make sure you're feeding your body with things that make it feel refreshed, fueled, and strong!

Chapter 20

THE WILDER WAY

(Mansplained for Men, by a Man)

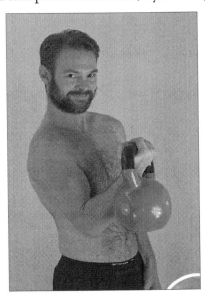

By Jack Wilder

OKAY, SO YOUR WIFE BOUGHT THIS BOOK, AND SUDDENLY SHE'S talking about "carb cycling" and "the Wilder Way," and black plates and white plates and gray plates, and suddenly Coke is evil and donuts are bad (but let's be honest, guys, we've always known they're bad, we just stopped caring), and now there's no Coke in the house, and you can't have carbs on Tuesdays because, for some stupid reason, she's decided Tuesdays are low-carb days, but then Wednesday she's giving you all sorts of carbs BUT NOTHING HAS CHEESE IN IT, and . . .

What the fuck, right?

And I'm also going to guess that she just shoved the book (or the eReader) into your hands and said "READ THIS . . . RIGHT NOW!", and so you're reading, but you're still scratching your head and wondering why you should give a crap about any of this. And you're thinking—even if you'd never actually SAY it to your wife in so many words, because you happen to like your balls attached thank you very much—that you like what you like, and you see no reason to change and if she won't give you the foods you like you'll get 'em yourself while you're out. Sneak in some McD's on the way home from work, or a slice of pizza at lunch, or grab a Coke at the gas station when you're pumping gas, or chow down a burger while you're at the bar with the guys.

What if I told you (cue the stern Morpheus glare and dramatic pause) . . . that you could STILL HAVE most of that? It won't be EXACTLY the same, but it'll still be burgers, still be pizza, still be beer, even cheesecake, brownies, pasta, all that. Donuts too.

No, I'm not going to sell you an eating plan. No, there's nobody you have to call or email, no auto-subscribe spam email lists, no apps to download, no calories to count, no meetings your wife is going to drag you to, no pre-packaged microwaveable plasticky low-fat bull-shit diet meals.

No, you're not going on a low-carb diet, and you're not going paleo or ketogenic, nor are you going on a 30-day all-shake juice cleanse diet.

THIS IS *NOT* A DIET.

Did you catch that, gentlemen? This thing, this weird "Wilder Way" your wife is doing is NOT a diet.

Well, let me go back and clarify. If you google "diet definition" right now, the following will pop up as the first definition: "the kinds of food that a person, animal, or community habitually eats." That's all a diet is. So yes, in that sense, it *is* a diet, in that it's the kinds of food you're eating. But it's not a diet in the second definition sense: "a special course of food to which one restricts oneself, either to lose weight or for medical reasons." It's *not* that.

Why?

Because my wife, who developed this Wilder Way, has tried every single diet known to mankind, and none of them ever worked. The weight never stayed off. No one can stick with a diet indefinitely, because 99.9% of so-called "diets" are just unsustainable, and most of them are just plain old medically unsound.

Why?

There are entire books dedicated to this subject, so I'm just going to do a quick and dirty crash course for you. Ready?

Diets are bullshit.

Your body REQUIRES carbs to function normally, so a no-carb/low-carb diet is just going to fail and even make you feel worse. Even if you lose weight initially, the moment you start eating carbs again—which is inevitable, because carbs are delicious—WHOOOOOP! The weight comes right back on, and usually with compound interest.

Then there's the good old standby diet: don't eat as much.

Also complete bullshit. You're meant to eat. Your body, once again, REQUIRES food, for . . . you know . . . everything. Like, for example, *being alive*, and not acting like a hangry monster all the damn time. Do I need to make that any simpler? I mean, it seems obvious. Yeah, you'll lose weight if you all eat every day is two leaves, four grains of rice, a sliver of lean turkey, and a glass of water. But you'll get hangry, and then you'll get . . . I don't know what to call it, rage-hangry? Whatever it's called when you haven't eaten for two days all you can think about is food and you feel like a Hungry Hungry Hippo version of The Incredible Hulk. And then, assuming you make it that long without eating, one of two things will happen: either you'll cave and binge-eat, or you'll pass out from malnutrition, end up in the hospital, and find yourself saddled with a massive bill. So that's out, too. Because it's stupid.

There are lots of other diets out there, which I see no reason to list and debunk one by one—because, as I said, there are entire books written by people with PhDs that will do a better job at it. But these diets are all the same, and the results are always the same.

The basic premise of human nutrition is very, very simple. You need three basic food groups for your body to function properly: carbohydrates, protein, and fats. And yes, you do need all three; you just need them in the right proportion, and you need the right kinds of each.

Let's talk carbs first, because those always get a bad rap. For a more in depth discussion of this topic, read the rest of this book, and even go back and read the first one, *Big Girls Do It Running*, because my wife is smarter than I am and explains this whole thing in better detail. I'm writing this chapter as a kind of hook, I guess. A chapter written by a guy who's gone through the same process you're going through. Read the first paragraph in this chapter again—yeah, that was me, except there was no book to read, just my wife trying a bunch of weird stuff I didn't understand.

So, carbs. Bread and pasta, yeah? That's pretty much it, right? What other carbs are there? Potatoes, for one. Rice. Broccoli, and the other fibrous greens your mom and/or dad made you eat when you were a kid. Quinoa—if you've never heard of it—is just another grain kind of like a mix between rice and pasta, and it's pronounced "Keen-WA," which I know just sounds pretentious as all hell, but regardless of how it's pronounced, it's pretty damn tasty when prepared right.

So, why do people go on low-carb diets, if we need carbs? What's wrong with bread and potatoes? Well, nothing, exactly. It's just that the modern American diet is pretty much ALL carbs, with a heaping portion of high-fat sauces and high-fat red meat. Think about it. Go to Olive Garden, and what's the first thing you get? White bread, slathered in butter. And then you order the four cheese Ziti, which is more bleached-flour white pasta, with heavy red sauce, and a metric shit-ton of cheese. It's absolutely delicious, and has so many carbs and so many calories in it that you might as well go to McDonald's and eat three double Quarter Pounder meals in a row, extra large drink and fries included. This is an exaggeration, obviously, but not by as much as you might think. This book is not about counting calories, and I couldn't begin to tell you how many calories are in those meals, either.

The point is, think about all those carbs. And, more accurately, the KIND of carbs. The white flour that goes into the bread and pasta is made from, to put it plainly, poison. That's NOT an exaggeration, unfortunately. Worse, that white flour hits your stomach and then your digestive system gets hold of it, and you know what it does? It turns all that flour to sugar. That is a 100% true, verifiable fact. THAT's why carbs are bad, guys. You eat three baskets of those damned delicious breadsticks at Olive Garden, and your body turns those breadsticks into sugar. And that sugar is going to do one of two things: either it's going to get burned off, or it's going to stick to your belly and clog up your arteries. Beer belly? Nah, son, that's a BREAD belly.

There's good news, though. There is bread you can eat that doesn't turn into sugar. And no, I don't mean the poop-brown cardboard "health food" crap you could build a pyramid out of. This bread is called sprouted whole grain, and it's actually amazing. Soft, tasty, good with peanut butter, or lunch meat, or even in the occasional grilled cheese. You can buy sprouted whole grain bread, sprouted whole grain pasta, rice . . . there are even healthy versions of things like pancake and waffle mix. No lie, I eat thick-ass Belgian waffles made with sprouted whole grain flour with syrup at least once a week. WITH BACON.

The difference is that the waffles are made from batter using nut and oats flours rather than processed and bleached wheat flour, and the syrup is made from stevia—a sweetener made from a plant. Stevia is not just a healthy sweetener, it's also highly concentrated so you need less of it—and the bacon is chicken bacon. I know, I know, non-pork bacon is anathema, but chicken bacon is, I swear, just as good as regular bacon. Better than turkey bacon, by far. Chicken bacon crisps up more like regular bacon, and has a very similar texture and flavor, and is a lot healthier for you than the pork version *or* the turkey bacon, which I call liar strips.

Have I got your interest yet?

I think I've skipped one important question I know a lot of you are asking: WHY SHOULD I CARE ABOUT EATING HEALTHY IN THE FIRST PLACE?

Um, so you live longer? So you don't get adult onset diabetes? So you can be there for your family?

The percentage of adults who develop diabetes is absolutely staggering, gentlemen. Look it up—there are probably figures on it in this book, or in the first one. My great-grandmother had diabetes, and my father developed it late in life, so I've seen it. It's not fun, and it CAN happen to you, and WILL, if you don't quit eating poisonous bullshit.

Need more reasons? Okay, I've got 'em. Everybody wants to lose weight and be stronger, right? Get those visible abs, bigger guns, a trimmer waist, boulder shoulders . . . all that. But maybe you've let yourself go a little, maybe you've got a spare tire—or two—around your midsection, and you don't remember the last time you ran any farther than from your car to the front door of the mall because it was raining. God knows, you might have big arms, but that shit ain't muscle. Yeah, I'm talking to you. I'm talking to myself, too. That was me. I had a growing belly, flabby arms, weak legs, no muscle, no energy.

And then I took a magic pill and it all melted away overnight, right?

Wrong, obviously. I didn't go soft overnight, and I won't get hard and strong again overnight either, and neither will you. There's no magic to this. No secret. No miracle pill. But if you want to lose the excess weight and put on muscle and get those abs visible and have energy, and possibly even see your various ailments fixed, this is the way forward.

Go to the front of this book and read the testimonials—none of those people were paid to write any of that. They're real, true, and honest results. Diabetes, Crohn's, and chronic back pain have been healed or made manageable, pounds and inches have been lost by the hundreds, clothing sizes have gone down, and their quality of life has improved.

Again, we're not selling anything except this book—which you already have in your hands. All you have to do is read it. Listen to your wife. Support her. Do this with her. And when you don't understand why you can't eat this or that, just go with it.

"But I don't like salad. Or veggies. Or sweet potatoes. Or salmon. Or avocado." Yeah, neither did I, and I wrote a chapter in this book on the subject of how your tastes WILL change. The same poisons in the food you've been eating that have clogged your arteries and turned to saggy fat have also dulled and trained your taste buds to only want those things. You know why? Because the "food" companies designed them intentionally so that you'd want more. This is no joke, and it's not an exaggeration. These companies know *exactly* what their "food-like product" is doing to your body, they just don't care . . . all they want is your money, so they design their products to be addictive.

Break the addiction. Eat the damn salad. It won't hurt you, and yes, you can put dressing on it, and have meat in it. I'm no advocate for a bowl of dry lettuce and a few bland carrots, because that's bullshit, if you ask me. Besides, neither you nor I are bunnies.

Yes, this requires change. It requires you to think about what you're eating, and when, and why. Yes, it means no more fast food, no more delivery pizza, no more Coke. But there are still burgers—just without the bun, which means you can actually eat MORE MEAT because you don't have that thick heavy bread filling you up. You can have pizza, and soda. Yes, real soda, in a wider variety of flavors than you can probably imagine.

There's also a section in this book with a few quick workouts, one for beginners, one intermediate, and one that's more advanced and challenging. How many pushups, sit-ups, and squats can you do right now? Right this very moment? Put the book down, shove the coffee table or your office chair out of the way, get down on the floor, and do pushups until you can't do any more, and then do sit-ups until you can't do any more, and then do squats until you can't do anymore.

Did you run out of breath and energy before your muscles actually gave out? Is the number embarrassingly low? Are you thinking about how many you used to be able to do in high school or college?

Can you run three miles? Try. Lace on those old Aasics sitting in the garage gathering dust, put on a pair of gym shorts and a T-shirt, and go out and start jogging. If you can't make it to the corner without huffing and puffing and feeling like you might die, then guess what? You're absolutely normal. That's most of America, guys.

You're meant for more. You're designed for more. You're made for strength. Your body is engineered to lift heavy loads, to pull weight, to run, to jump. Right now, though, your body is clogged and weak and soft. Because you've been eating garbage. I know this, because I was clogged and weak and soft from eating garbage. Within a couple months of this new lifestyle, I was doing pushups and pull-ups and sit-ups and squats and running three or six miles several times a week, and deadlifting nearly 300 pounds and benching nearly my own weight. And I'm not trying to be a bodybuilder or a runner. I just learned to love moving, I learned to love challenging myself. I LOVE the feeling of finishing a killer workout and being totally smoked. I finish a hard run, and my legs are shaky and I can't breathe, but I feel like a badass.

Maybe you do lift, maybe you can bench me plus another fifty pounds, maybe you can back squat half a dozen 45 plates or even more . . . but you know you have a layer of pudge covering those muscles. You have the muscles, you have the strength, it's just . . . buried, hidden. Maybe you play hockey or football or baseball in a men's rec league, but you're just not as fast as you used to be, you don't have the endurance you once did . . .

Guess what? Eat the right foods in the right proportion, quit eating processed garbage and bleached flour and quit drinking a liquid that can *dissolve metal* (Coke). You know what will happen? That extra fluff will melt away. Those muscles you already have will start to pop, your shape will taper to that killer wedge, you'll be able to lift more and run faster and for longer. It's not magic, it's not a gimmick, it's just the incredible power of clean eating.

Give it a try. What do you have to lose? Give this book, this Wilder Way, a few months. Stick with it, give the foods you're not sure about a few chances. More importantly, if your wife shoved this book in your hands and demanded you read this chapter, just give *her* a chance, and give her your support. Chances are, she wants you to try this with her because she wants you to be healthier. She already loves you and is attracted to you—she married you, after all—but what do you think will happen if you lose weight and gain muscle and have energy and power and stamina?

Yeah, *that*. A *lot* more of it. Trust me on this one. Sexual performance—stamina, testosterone level, and refractory period—is directly tied to proper nutrition. All that will get better too. Which makes her happy, which in turns means *more* of it . . . I swear I'm not making this up or just blowing smoke up your ass. It's real, and I'm living proof of it.

Point is, just give it a try.

Chapter 21:

BALANCE: FINDING IT AND KEEPING IT!

"Women in particular . . . need to do a better job of putting
ourselves higher on our own 'to do' list."
—Michelle Obama

JUST TODAY, A WOMAN MESSAGED ME TO TELL ME THAT ALTHOUGH she loved all of my books and had lost 40 pounds on the #WilderWay she wouldn't be buying this book. When I asked her why, she explained that there was just no way that she could add one more thing to her schedule. She said she was a mom, and she had hobbies and too many other things to take up more exercise.

I spent a half hour talking with her and explaining that I am exactly the same. I'm a mom, wife, and businesswoman, and I own a farm with over 100 animals. I have very little time for long, grueling workouts. In fact, if anything, this book is a way for you and I to spend even LESS time in the gym or running, and spend more time with those beautiful kids and that sexy hubby. I don't want to make life harder for either of us! I really hope to make things easier.

Balance is hard. I know this. I think I could write an entire book on women in America discovering the importance of balance. I think balance is critical for finding and holding onto your joy, right? You can't be a good mom unless you have some time for yourself. You can't be a good wife if you don't sleep at night. You can't perform well at work when you feel like crap all of the time. All of these things are connected.

I know it isn't just a few of us who struggle to be everything to everyone each and every day. Especially if you are a working mama, I know that just finding a few minutes each week to run or lift weights might be a big ask. I totally understand and empathize because I often feel the same way.

What has really helped me is to focus on my greatest goals in life. What is the legacy I want to leave for my family and my children? First, I want my kids to have two parents as long as possible. I know that beyond anything else in the world, my husband wants me here with him. As cliché as it sounds, we really hope to grow old together. I want to see my husband dance with our daughter at her wedding. I want to play with my grandkids. I want to spend as many moments as I can on this earth with those I love, and I bet you feel the same way. This means my health has to be a top priority.

We can push healthy living aside and put it on the back burner. But, eventually, something will pop up, like a diabetes diagnosis, dangerously high blood pressure, or even cancer. But really, our quality of life is up to us. We might not know when we will take our last breath, but we can decide how we want to feel between now and then.

Doesn't it seem like everyone has stress piled on top of anxiety with a side of depression? I think this has to do with balance, too. We're always rushing around, yet we're always sitting down; we don't get outside, and we don't have the time to move or to exercise; we're bored so we endlessly scroll on social media looking for who knows what—I think all of this can even contribute to anxious hunger. What really helps me is consciously trying to slow down.

Really, really, slow down. Spend a few minutes just breathing. Have you tried some yoga? You can download free apps that have great little routines that only take a few minutes. Spending 2% of your day just slowing down is often passed over in favor of other things. But we never question the hour or two spent mindlessly scrolling on our phones, or watching something on TV that really doesn't get us closer to our goals and what we really want from life.

I know this can be a hard cycle to break. Jack and I have had to make changes to ensure that we have this time and this balance in our lives. It isn't really that we need more time in the day—it's that we need to make better use of the time we have. It becomes too easy to become lazy about self-care because we think we will eventually be less busy and have more time. Let's just be honest and say we won't ever have that. And if we do, it will probably be the day we die.

Be honest with yourself about your goals. What do you really want, and what might you have to change, or adjust to have that? Can you find half an hour for a walk around the block? Maybe you always wanted to try a dance class, or maybe you could find some peace and enjoyment with art. Whatever it is, I believe in sitting down and figuring out what you want. Enjoy it, and find joy in your life. These things are critically important. Make a conscious choice to find balance and keep it.

How am I working to find my balance?

Maybe sharing more of my focus with you might help you to figure out what are the most important things for you. My relationship with my husband and children are some of my greatest goals. I want those to be strong. I want them to be intentional. I never want my husband or kids to think they aren't important to me. So, how do

I do that? Well, I had to figure out the things that best expressed this to my family. I know my daughter loves it when I spend time playing just with her. My little boys want lots of stories before bed. My kids want us to pray together before school. My husband needs lots of sex. This is my list and my life!

When you can identify your own things and really focus on them, you can hopefully let go of some of the other things that maybe aren't as important in the day to day.

Maybe you can reorganize the to-do list, or maybe the list can get shorter.

I really believe in routine and schedules. Not only do kids feel secure when they can count on structure, but I find this works for adults, too. I've worked out of a planner for years and it is big and ugly, but it helps keep me organized. I also have lists in places where I won't forget before going into the next room. I keep lists on my phone, on the pantry door, and on post-it notes in my office. Whatever you need to do to stay on task and organized will help. Plan out your day so you can be more effective. Work smarter, not harder.

Take some time at the start of the day to assess what's ahead, and again at the end of the day to to examine what you've done. What did you not get done? What needs to happen tomorrow? What can you let go of and no longer worry about? For me, the ONLY way this happens is if my phone is away from me; if the phone is close, I'll start working the moment I wake up until the moment I fall asleep. That is just my nature.

Jack and I made the decision to have times in our day that are "phone free." We don't use phones during dinner or until after the kids to go bed. We check for any emergencies after the kids are in bed and then the phones go back on chargers so we can spend some time focused on each other, or just relaxing without the pressure of the phone.

I promise, if you start charging your phone in another part of your home, you will eventually forget about it. Some of my favorite moments of the day are when Jack and I have phone-free time. No, that isn't even what I mean! Get your mind out of the gutter.

Really though, these moments are the ones you will remember and treasure. You deserve some hands-on time with your spouse and kids. This will absolutely help you find that balance, I promise. Just try it. There are very good things happening away from your tablet, phone, or computer . . . unless you're reading one of my books. If that's what you're doing, forget everything I just said.

Lastly, and as I move into my next chapter, I think something that moms especially need to do is treat themselves. Now listen, I'm not saying you need to take a tropical vacation by yourself, but you should allow yourself to relax and enjoy life. Have that piece of chocolate and glass of wine without guilt. Get a pedicure if that makes you feel good. Go out for a girls' night or lunch. Relationships are important in finding balance, and your relationship with yourself is the most important one you've got.

If you are down a few sizes on my plan, go out and find an outfit that really makes you feel good. Maybe you don't have money for something new? Put out a shout on Facebook that you are looking for something in a certain size. I've found especially in my group that woman love to bless each other in this way. Maybe you have a friend who's a similar size who might let you come play dress up in her closet. Add some wine and a snack and you've got quite a party right there!

Don't underestimate the importance of good, genuine friendships. Invest in those because often close friends are the ones who can call you out when you're running yourself ragged, and they can help you get back to balance. So tonight, forget about that to-do list of a hundred things and write down the things that are the most important to you today and focus your day around those things.

One day at a time. This is a marathon, not a sprint.

PRO TIP: Try to put all of your energy and focus on the things you can control, and let go and trust in God for the things you can't. Sometimes the dishes and laundry seem more important than they really are; spend your time on what is truly important first. I promise the dishes and laundry will wait for you. Making sure you're rested and refreshed is more important . . . unless you're literally down to your last pair of pants. If it's a choice between taking a half hour for yourself and wearing clean pants, you probably should do some laundry. ☺

Chapter 22

HEALTH AND WELLNESS: FACTS VS FICTION

EVERY SINGLE DAY ON MY *BIG GIRLS DO IT RUNNING* Facebook group, I hear health myths that I want to try and explain and debunk. These are health urban legends that just don't seem to die. We need to stop listening to these myths and try to stick to the facts. Don't sweat the small stuff, and when you fall off plan a bit, jump back on.

- "Muscle weighs more than fat."
  - o **False**: Muscle and fat weigh the same; muscle just takes up less space. Also, weight doesn't necessarily drop at the same moment you are building up muscle. Both the building of muscle and loss of weight take time. Just be patient.

- "Eating eggs causes high cholesterol."
  - o **False**: Eating eggs won't cause high cholesterol. Poor diet, fried and packaged foods, obesity, lack of exercise, smoking, and diabetes is what causes high cholesterol.

- "Honey and agave are good for you."
  - o **False**: Honey is yummy, yes—I remember, as a child, eating a big, white fluffy biscuit with loads of butter and honey. Honey and agave both raise blood sugar. I don't believe these things are good for you, and I don't recommend them.

- "Carbohydrates make you fat."
  - o **False**: Not all carbohydrates are the same. Please go back and read my chapter on carbohydrates. They have really gotten a bad rep and we need to promote healthy carbs, especially to our kids, who really need them to grow healthy and strong.

- "You shouldn't eat at night."
  - o **False:** I've seen nothing to support this. Nada. If you need a snack after dinner, eat it.

- "Food allergies cause weight gain."
  - o **False:** Allergies usually cause the opposite issue because your body wants to expel what it is allergic to. Food allergies are very real, but I've found more often that what people are actually allergic to is the way a food is processed vs the food itself. I have seen time and time again that my gluten-free friends can enjoy sprouted wheat, and my friends with nut and other similar issues have no problems with them once other toxins are out of the body. My suggestion is to proceed with caution and always continue a conversation with your doctor about your allergies and how to treat them within your eating plan.

- "Lifting weights will make women look like men."
  - o **False**: Nope, no way! Women who compete in bodybuilding work day and night to achieve that muscle mass and low body fat percentage. Lifting a kettlebell a few days a week is not going to make you look like a muscle-bound dude, but it WILL tone muscle, shape your body, and burn away fat.

- "You have to eat five small meals a day to lose weight," or, "You should only eat three meals a day to lose weight." Or "only eat a certain boxed, pre-portioned amount", or "only drink shakes".
  - o **NO, NO, NO!** Eat when you're hungry. Eat real food. You don't need to count calories, macros, berries, or grains. This is such a waste of time, friends. Focus on the quality of your food and how you feel. Get out of the mind trap—it's all false.

- "You need to spend an hour doing cardio five days a week to be fit."
  - o **Baloney:** You do not need to do this. The science just doesn't support it. Find a physical activity that you enjoy. Sprint for 20 minutes, lift weights, walk, jog, dance, play soccer. Even 10 minutes each day will improve your cardiovascular health. Just get that body moving and you'll be healthier and more fit each day!

- "Gluten- free food is healthier than regular food."
  - o **False:** Gluten-free doesn't necessarily mean healthier, and if you're talking about packaged foods it can even

mean it has more sugar, as well as fillers like corn and soy, not to mention lots of chemicals. My advice is to keep an eye on these labels and really try to stick to foods with minimal ingredients in whole-food form that you recognize and can pronounce.

- "Running is bad for your knees."
  - o **False:** A Stanford University study found that older runners' knees were no less healthy than those of people who don't run. Lifting weights and strength training a few times a week will help you build muscle, strengthen your bones and joints, and lower chances of injury.

- "Sleep has nothing to do with overall health."
  - o **False:** Studies have shown that women who don't get at least seven hours of sleep each night weigh more than those who do. Get your sleep in and rest fully. For your body to function properly, it's important to rest.

Chapter 23

ABOVE ALL, LOVE YOURSELF

BEAR WITH ME FOR A CHAPTER, BECAUSE I'M GOING TO GET A BIT mom on you and maybe even a little mushy. This chapter might be long, and it might even get preachy.

I grew up as a very fat kid. I think I was about eight when I was first classified as morbidly obese. Nothing ever worked for me. I spent at least half of my childhood crying myself to sleep at night asking God why he had afflicted me in this way. As a child, it always felt like something was very wrong with me. I never felt normal or okay. Glaring eyes were always on me. As a result, my character and personality really had to over-compensate because without getting laughs or positive reactions from my peers in some way, I don't think I would have survived. It has taken me a very, very long time to learn to love myself. To cherish myself. To take care of myself. It still hurts today, at 37, for me to even think about it too deeply.

I'm sure that many people probably think that my program is too restrictive, or over the top with the elimination of most of the products found in your local store. I'm sure people say things behind my back about how I'm missing out, or how I'm cruel to my kids because they don't get to partake in the "normal kid foods and treats."

Let me explain what I think this program really is. The Wilder Way is a love-yourself program. It's a program based on putting only the best foods into your body. It's a program about taking the time and energy to really care for your body through nutrition and movement. If there is ANYTHING I want you to take away from this book, it's that you deserve this. You deserve to feel whole, healthy, and strong. I do, and so do you. I'll even take it step farther and say that this is your moment to finally have that. What would make you feel truly healthy? What would you need to be capable of feeling really strong? Let's take the first steps to make that happen today. Friends, this might not happen overnight, or even in a few months. But if you do this more and more, day by day, little by little, I promise you that you'll begin to see and feel things you may have never thought possible. You will run that full mile, lift that barbell, hike the mountain, and see test results from your doctor that say you are in fact HEALTHY! This is something I want for you *so* badly.

There is only one thing that can keep you from this, only one person who will keep telling you that this isn't possible, that you won't ever be strong, or learn to eat healthy, or control the cravings, or give up the soda, or lift the heavy weight, or run the mile and that's ... you, yourself, and your own doubts. Listen, I know that bitch too! Her voice is a powerful thing.

Let me tell you what I've learned so far, and what I know to be true:

YOU ARE STRONGER. You are unstoppable. I know you've had years of pain. Maybe it's all emotional, but maybe it is also that your body is just tired. You have sore and bad knees? You have asthma? Your back hurts? You don't have time? You just aren't smart enough?

That's me! I am all of of those things. Yet, I did it. I'm here nine years after being told I probably had cancer. I've been unable to get out of bed. I've had to have a home health nurse come daily to take care of me and give me life-saving infusions. Yet, here I am! Healthy for the very first time in my life. Running, lifting, walking, and wogging!

This isn't just a miracle, or an answer to a prayer, friends. This is science: Sugar + the human body = slow death. So, I want to talk to you as frankly as I can. I want to change the conversation that might be going on in your head right now.

You CAN do this. You CAN be strong and healthy.

If you hear yourself saying, "I could never lift this weight," say instead, "One day I will be able to lift this weight," and then go grab a smaller one, I don't even care if it's a two-pound dumbbell! Just keep lifting until you have that down, and it becomes easy, and then grab a heavier one!

If you hear yourself saying, "I'm weak," instead say, "I was made to be strong, and every single day I am getting better and stronger."

If the voice in your head keeps saying that you have no will power and you will never reach your goals because there is no way you can ever change, then I want you to say out loud to yourself that you WILL reach these goals. Each meal is an opportunity to make healthier choices, and each day is an opportunity to use your body.

Let me be honest and say I don't think you will ever really be super excited to work out as soon as you wake up in the morning. I actually question the sanity of people who wake up feeling that way, but I promise that you will get to the point where you will both want it and need it. Being good to your body with movement and exercise (yes, even just walking) will become a kind of therapy, not only for your body, but also for your mind. You *will* start to feel stronger and better just by putting that first foot in front of the other.

And now the big one—if the voice in your head tells you that you don't deserve this, that for some reason you don't deserve full health or the use of your body in the way God intended, I want you to say with me . . . I want you tell that voice to **FUCK OFF**! I truly believe that the feeling of not being worthy is at the root of why we give up on our journey to health, often before we even get started.

I hear all the time how five days into my program someone gained three pounds and so they've decided that this just isn't going to work for them and so they're giving up, they're throwing in the towel. *REALLY*? Do you *really* think you're only worth a week or two? Please ladies, please give yourself the gift of time and grace. You need to learn to love yourself every day. Change won't happen overnight.

Ironically, I just saw a People magazine cover where Oprah was once again saying she had finally made her peace with food. Gosh, I really hope she has but, as I've learned along my journey, often we think our health issues have more to do with our failings than it actually does. Eighty percent of your health issues have to do with the junk you've been told is food. This isn't about you! This is about companies wanting to make as much money as possible. Don't take that crap—it's bullshit, and it isn't about you. Once you get back to real food, nutritious food not filled with sugar and processed chemicals, you'll actually find that so much of the rollercoaster you've been on had nothing to do with you at all, but with the fake, evil *NOT*-food shit you've been sold. I'm asking you to do a total 180 in every thought you've ever had about food.

Stop the conversation in your head now, *please!*

As I mentioned earlier in the book, a few months ago I realized I was having issues with body dysmorphia, and it was expressing itself in weird ways. I just didn't feel "normal size." What did normal size mean anyway? I couldn't figure out my body, or really get comfortable in it—not in the ways I should have been. I just felt awkward. The excess skin was bothering me. I couldn't shop at the stores I had shopped at before. I was trying to figure out how to get accustomed to the person I saw in the mirror. She's different in some ways, but she's also the same.

This is hard to explain to someone who hasn't been through these sorts of drastic body transformations, but the strange phase of rediscovery and pain is a very normal part of the process. Yes, there's joy, but there is also grief—grief over the time I lost as an unhealthy, young woman, grief that I didn't learn these things earlier, shame at the state of my body, shame from the abuse of my body. It's pretty complicated when you've lived the majority of your life in a body that was not only unhealthy, but is a reminder of emotional and physical pain.

I was also angry with myself for even having these issues in the first place. I had waited all my life to have a healthy body and now I was dealing with these stupid mental and emotional hang-ups. I finally decided I should probably talk to a professional; it was time to make friends with my body. Yes, it wasn't in the shape or size I had always envisioned, but it had gotten me this far, and it had given me my beautiful children. I made an appointment with a therapist to discuss the best ways to go about shifting my mental and emotional processes, and I think what I learned might help you a bit, too.

I learned several things when I sat down and began talking to Dr. E, my therapist.

First, I learned that I needed to change the way I thought about my body, the way I looked at my body, and make some peace with that. My body will always have extra skin, lumpy cellulite (I'm convinced all the fat left has been here since 1984 and won't leave), I am covered in scars, my feet will always be big, my bottom half and my top half probably won't ever match. There, I said it to you too, so it's really out there.

Now, here's the other side of the truth: although I have lots of skin, my body is much healthier than it ever was before. The skin might be a reminder of where I have been, but as long as it's hanging it's a reminder of where I'll never be again. That lumpy cellulite ain't pretty, but very few people see it. There are so many worse afflictions, or more painful things to bear. My scars tell a story, a story with a hero in it, and even though the hero is tattered, she's also me. These big feet have carried me across finish line after finish line. God has blessed me with a husband who has no problem with my bottom.

Seriously though, I'm learning to accentuate those things with my fashion choices and I'm lucky that stores like New York & Company, American Eagle, and Fashion Nova make so many great, inexpensive clothes for my body type. Remember ladies—just because the dress fits, doesn't mean you have to own it . . . there are so many options out there for us now.

Here's another thing that shocked me when I talked to Dr. E: she asked me if I thought I had a normal-sized body, and I immediately said no. My response wasn't something I really even thought about. What *is* normal these days anyway? I think, in America, the current average size for women is 14-16, so I'm actually a bit below that, yet I still FELT so much bigger. My body just didn't identify any other way, probably because most of my life I was always the biggest person in the room.

It is at the root of my psyche to just feel *big*.

I've realized I have to give myself grace and time with this. It's okay that I'm still getting used to this new body; I haven't lived inside a space this size since 6th or 7th grade, so this will not happen overnight. We can't snap our fingers and immediately adapt to the new normal. It's still hard for me not to ask for a seatbelt extender, or not push my car seat all the way back before I get in. It's hard to remember that I don't need the largest size anymore, and I don't need to pay the extra fee to have something made even bigger. This is how things were MY WHOLE LIFE. We can't expect our minds to adjust at the same rate as our bodies.

As a person who always tries to challenge and push herself, this is hard for me to talk about. I've been abused, and I've treated myself badly and beat myself up so many times in my life. But this is a new day, and I am going to let the emotional healing happen on the time-line it needs. I know that acknowledging this and continuing to work on it will only help, and I hope my sharing helps you, too.

The way I've decided to approach it actually has two parts. First, I'm being kind to my body. I am looking in the mirror and focusing on every single good thing I can see. I'm taking LOTS of full body photos of myself. If you were to look back through my photos over the years, you would see that I have almost no full body photos. I don't even think I used to look at my body below my neck when I looked at myself in the mirror. Now, I try to take a moment and really look at myself. I want you to try and do that too—really see yourself, really feel yourself. Don't just take a short glimpse, but take a really good, loving look. I'm not sure this is something we are ever really taught to do, and maybe we should talk to our daughters about it, too.

- This is a tiny commercial for the *BIG GIRLS DO IT RUNNING COMPANION JOURNAL*. Journaling has helped me SO MUCH! There are many times that writing down measurements, recording accomplishments, or just journaling my feelings has made all of the difference in this journey. I really suggest getting a journal to write down some of these thoughts and feelings so you can look back and see how far you've really come.

Above all, I think positive self-talk and positive self-action are the most important pieces of this puzzle. Still, even years into this journey, I'll slip into negative self-talk. My oh-so helpful husband will say to me, "J, what would you say if one of the ladies in your group said something like that about herself? Would you let her talk that way? No? Well then, don't let yourself do it either!" Gosh, Jack isn't always right but when he is, he REALLY is.

So I'm telling myself what I tell you: be proud not only of where you are now, but where you came from. Be proud of each and every step on this journey. We will grow, we will be stronger, and we will run on together.

Say it with me:

I'm working toward a better, healthier me.
I deserve to feel good!
I am going to love myself.
I will work to love myself exactly as I am today.
I will talk and think positively about myself.
My body is beautiful.

The Wilder Way 2.0

MOVEMENT CHALLENGE

Try to increase both workouts and healthy food choices
each week as best you can!
Our goal is clean, mean, and lean!

Jack says: "This is where we talk about my big, heavy bells. I'm
talking about kettlebells, people, get your minds out of the gutter!"

In this chapter, we get down to the business of strength training. As
you will see, we have a daily plan that will take you through the entire
week. Each day, you have the option of doing Beginner, Intermediate,
or Advanced workouts. Along with the training details, I've indicat-
ed the best food plan for each day.

Just like the 8-week challenge in *BIG GIRLS DO IT RUNNING*,
don't freak if you don't lose pounds or inches right away. Strength
training will provide a big change in the body, so just give yourself
time and make sure to record your progress. We are in this together.
Slow and steady!

MONDAY

NUTRITION: WHITE PLATE DAY

Three meals and three snacks today—CARBS AND PROTEINS in each meal and snack.

Little to no fats at all!

WORKOUT: 40 minutes of weightlifting and cardio (this is what I call a "heavy" day)

Beginner Workout:

1. Warm up: One mile of walking/wogging or running as fast as you can. It's okay to stop as needed, just push yourself and get that heart rate up.
2. Pick **3–4** of these basic strength movements and rotate daily. Yes, you can modify these if needed! Set a timer and see how fast you can do the movements, and try to beat your best times. If these numbers start to feel too easy and you are getting through the workout really fast, just add more sets or increase the number you are doing for each exercise.

   - 25 jumping jacks
   - 20 pushups or sit-ups
   - 1-minute plank/30 second side plank
   - 12 lunges to the back or side (6 on each leg)
   - 15 squats or 10 jump squats
   - 10 straight leg lifts
   - 1-minute wall sit
   - 30 second sprints
   - 25 high knees

- 15 hip thrusts
- 20 butterfly kicks
- 20 mountain climbers (10 each leg)
- 1 minute of jumping rope

Intermediate workout:

1. Warm up: 60 jumping jacks or walking jacks. (As an aside on warm ups: always do some kind of warm up before beginning a workout to get your heart beating, your muscles stretched and heated, and your mind in workout mode; warm-ups shouldn't smoke you, but they *should* get you breathing a little hard).

2. 5 Sit-ups—no crunches, these are full sit-ups. Lie down with your back on the floor, feet pulled up near your butt, and extend your arms over your head parallel to the floor as if reaching for the wall behind you—*not* over your face as if reaching for the ceiling—and then sit up explosively while swinging your arms over your head to touch your toes, and then lie back down, swinging your arms back parallel with the floor. That's one rep.

3. 5 Pushups—modify as needed! If you can't do a classic standard pushup, put your knees on the ground.

4. 5 Air Squats—keep your spine straight, feet shoulder-width apart, lean forward and sit down over your feet; your shins should track over the top of your toes in a straight line. Try to get as far down as you can. As you stand up, imagine you are pushing the floor away with your feet while squeezing your butt cheeks together. For added balance and fun, pretend you're Bruce Lee and extend your arms as you squat down,

making a triangle with your index fingers and thumbs, palms facing away, and lower your arms on the way up.

RECAP: 5 Pushups, 5 Sit-ups, and 5 Squats—this is **ONE** set performed with as little rest as possible in between movements. After each set, rest 1–3 minutes as needed, and then do another set. Try to do five sets in total.

Post-workout Cardio: Run one half-mile at top comfortable speed; record your time and try to beat it every time you workout.

Advanced workout:

If you can, get a kettlebell for this workout. You just need one—a 15 or 20 lb bell to start with is perfect—but a dumbbell will work too. You don't HAVE to have a kettlebell to be successful, but it is great to have. Check your local big box store, or a sporting goods store, as they are often on sale. Amazon has lots of great low cost options, too!

1. Warm up: 60 jumping jacks.

2. 5 Military Presses (each side, if you're using a weight):

Hold the kettlebell in one hand in front of you, touching the center of your chest, then push it upward over your head, hold it at the top for a second or two, and then slowly lower it down. Switch hands, and repeat.

If you don't have a weight available, then do the bodyweight modification: feet flat on the floor, touch your palms to the floor in front of your toes and walk your hands forward four or five pac-es, so your butt is sticking up in the air—the downward-facing dog position for you yoga people—now lower your head to the ground between your hands and push yourself back up, keeping your core tight and your legs as straight as possible. This is one rep.

3.(5) Bent Rows:

If you have a kettlebell or dumbbell, hold it in one hand, bend at the waist with your back straight and knees slightly bent. Extend the weight toward the ground beneath your chest, pull it up and backward toward your hip, then return it to the extended position. This is one rep.

If you don't have a weight, this will work with just about any number of household objects, such as a gallon of milk or juice, or a small carry-on size suitcase or duffel bag filled with a few books.

The 5 presses and the 5 rows are done one after the other without resting between; this is called a superset. Do at least three sets of five each of rows and presses—and no, it doesn't matter which order you do them in, but if the movement is something you do left side and then right side, this means five *per side*. A superset means you'll do 5 rows and 5 presses, and then rest, 5 rows and 5 presses, and rest—that would be two sets. Anywhere I say "superset," this is what I mean.

4.5 Goblet Squats:

If you are using a weight, hold it in both hands in front of your chest, elbows tucked in against your sides. Do a squat, holding the weight at chest level. Like with the regular squats described above, keep your spine straight and flat and lean forward a little as you squat so your weight stays centered over your feet. Try to go as low as you can before rising back up. This is called a Goblet Squat. If you don't have a weight, just do 10 air squats as described in the intermediate workout.

5.5 Alternating Lunges—this means five on each leg, so 10 total:

Holding the weight like you did for the Goblet Squat, take a step forward and touch your back knee to the floor, then return to standing and do the same with the other leg. This is one rep.

As with the upper body movements, the Goblet Squats and Alternating Lunges are done together as a superset, so you do the squats, then the lunges, and then rest. Try for three sets.

6.15 Sit-ups, as described in the intermediate workout section:

Lie down with your back on the floor, feet pulled up near your butt, and extend your arms over your head parallel to the floor as if reaching for the wall behind you—*not* over your face as if reaching for the ceiling—and then sit up explosively while swinging your arms over your head to touch your toes, and then lie back down, swinging your arms back parallel with the floor. That's one rep.

7.15 Leg Raises:

Lie flat on the floor on your back, your arms at your sides. Then raise your feet, legs extended and knees locked, up and over your head as far as you can until your tailbone leaves the floor, and then lower them slowly. That's one rep. Don't let your feet touch the floor between repetitions.

If you need some help with this, grab onto a standing partner's calves, or hold onto a heavy weight, or anything that will work as some kind of counterbalance.

Hopefully by now you're seeing the pattern: as a Superset, do the Sit-Ups and Leg Raises one after the other with no rest. Then take a one- or two-minute break, or longer as needed, and do another set. Always take *at least* one-minute breaks between sets, and no more than three minutes. Try for three sets.

Last, but not least, run one mile at top speed, recording your time.

Advanced Workout Recap:
- 5 kettlebell/dumbbell military presses (or military press pushups) and 5 bent rows done as a superset; one set minimum, but try for three sets as a goal; rest 1–3 minutes between sets.
- 5 goblet squats and 5 alternating lunges done as a superset; one set minimum, but try for three sets as a goal; rest 1–3 minutes between sets.
- 5 sit-ups and 5 leg raises done as a superset; one set minimum, but try for three sets as a goal; rest 1–3 minutes between sets.
- one-mile run for time.

TUESDAY

NUTRITION: BLACK PLATE DAY
Three meals and two snacks—FATS AND PROTEINS in each meal and snack.

WORKOUT: This is a light workout day with 30 minutes of a dance video or light core work—very little to no lifting.

Do a dance fitness video, or run a 5K at an easy pace, or do 20 Burpees. A Burpee is deceptively simple: stand up straight, jump up and reach for the ceiling, then squat down, move into the pushup position, do a single pushup modified as needed, then either jump or walk your feet up between your palms, stand up, and jump again . . . this is ONE rep.

Basically, today's workout is anything that will get your heart beating and your body sweating. Playing tag with the kids counts, or jumping rope—Double Dutch, anyone? This is about keeping it simple and fun, so there's nothing specific for advanced workouts on light days. Just have fun, get moving, and challenge yourself! Ride a bike farther and faster than you normally might, swim laps, go to the ice rink or roller rink, skate around the block on your skates, or skateboard . . . you get the picture. Light workout days are about fun movements that challenge you to push your body. Planks, crunches or other core workouts are a great choice, too.

WEDNESDAY

NUTRITION: BLACK PLATE DAY
Three meals and two snacks—FATS AND PROTEINS in each meal and snack.

WORKOUT: This is a light workout day—30 minutes of a dance video or light core work, very little to no lifting.

Do something different than you did yesterday. Or do it for longer, or harder. If you did 20 burpees yesterday, try for 25 or 30—trust me, those extra few will really smoke you. Again, this is about keeping it simple and fun, so there's nothing specific for workouts on light days. Just have fun, get moving, and challenge yourself! Ride a bike, swim laps, skate around the block on your skates, or skateboard . . . you get the picture. Remember, light workout days are about fun movements that challenge you to push your body. Planks, crunches or other core workouts are a great choice, too.

THURSDAY

NUTRITION: WHITE PLATE DAY

Three meals and three snacks—CARBS AND PROTEINS at each meal and snack

Little to no fats at all!

WORKOUT: This is a heavy workout day—45 minutes of weight lifting and cardio

Beginner, intermediate, and advanced workouts: repeat the workout plan from Monday. Really focus on feeling each movement. Do the movements slowly and in control. Breathe in as you relax, breathe out as you do the work. So, for a push-up, breathe in on the way down, and breathe out on the way up. Keep your back straight, focus on the flex of each muscle as it contracts. Learn how your body responds, and if you need to take a break, take a break!

FRIDAY

NUTRITION: BLACK PLATE DAY

Three meals and two snacks – FATS AND PROTEINS at each meal and snack.

WORKOUT: This is a light workout day—30 minutes of a dance video or light core work – very little to no lifting.

This is the last real exercise day of the week, so really try to challenge yourself. If you ran three miles, try for three and a half or four, or try to complete the three miles in less time. Push yourself! You might hate me and yourself and life and everything while you're doing it, but when you're done, you'll feel like a beast!

SATURDAY

NUTRITION: BLACK PLATE DAY

Three meals and two snacks—FATS AND PROTEINS at each meal and snack.

WORKOUT: This is a light workout day. Run or walk with the family, or do dance videos for easy and fun cardio. This day is supposed to be light and easy, and not as challenging as the light days during the week.

SUNDAY

NUTRITION: GRAY ALL DAY!!!!

WORKOUT: REST and RELAX!

PRO TIP: If you have a husband or children who want to gain or maintain weight, then they should be doing gray plates all day every day.

ALTERNATE WORKOUTS

Listed below are some quick 15-minute options for when you want to spice up your workout, or don't have a lot of time. You can do these by themselves on days you're crunched for time, or if you're feeling *really* badass, do them at the end of another workout as a finisher. These are all going to be pretty challenging, but they are also adjustable, meaning if you can't do the workout as written then just do fewer reps or put less time on the clock.

The goal with any timed set is to really challenge yourself, really push your limits. It's only 15 minutes, so go hard! Go for that one last set! As always, be careful and use proper form with every movement to avoid injury, and listen to your body! If you feel like you're just done, then be done.

ALTERNATE WORKOUT #1

This workout should be done in 15 minutes, *excluding* the warm up.

1.Warm-up—60 jumping jacks

2.Set a timer for 15 minutes and do the following with as little rest between repetitions *and* sets as possible. Basically, you should be busting your ass as hard as you can for the entire 15 minutes (this goes for all three of these alternate workouts). Remember to focus on proper form for each movement

- Do as a set: 5 pushups, 5 sit-ups, and 5 squats—the 15 individual repetitions count as ONE set.

So: 5 pushups + 5 sit-ups + 5 squats = one set; see how many sets you can do in 15 minutes with as little rest as possible throughout. This is fun to do with a partner, as a competition . . . you can even set a friendly low-cost wager, e.g. the winner buys the loser a bottle of Josh Cab Sav, or a Lily's bar, or something like that. It's meant to be *fun*, so don't get crazy competitive with each other.

ALTERNATE WORKOUT #2

This workout uses a single kettlebell and should be done in 15 minutes, *excluding* the warm up.

1. Warm-up—60 jumping jacks
2. 3 Kettlebell Cleans, 2 Goblet Squats, 1 Military Press—you can also switch the number of reps and movement types around, so you do 1, 3, 2 respectively, or 2, 3,1, etc., but you always do the movements in that order.

What's a kettlebell clean? Simply put, you hold the bell in front of your chest like you're doing a press, but instead of lifting it overhead, fold forward at the waist and let it drop down in front of your thighs, hike it back between your legs, and then straighten your back by snapping your hips forward so the bell swings away, and then pull it up and in to return it to your chest.

Ugh—that sounds super complicated written out; really, it's not complicated at all, I promise! Type "kettlebell clean" into your internet search bar—a quick Google search of that term will bring up any number of tutorial videos, and Jasinda and I will be posting videos for these workouts as well in the Facebook group. Watch the video, try a few cleans as practice, and you'll get the hang of it. These are done on each side, so if you have one bell, three reps = three reps on the left *and* three on the right.

For the squat, do a Goblet Squat as described above.

The press is as described above as well: hold the bell in the rack position and press it up overhead, then lower it down to the rack.

When you do this 15 minute workout, do as many sets as possible. As a reminder, the three movements count together as one set, so 3 cleans + 2 squats + 1 press = one set. This particular set is called Armor Building, and credit for this killer programming goes to Pat Flynn from Breaking Muscle. Armor Building is an old standby for Jasinda and me, and it's great for when you're short on time and want to do something different and quick, yet still challenging.

ALTERNATE HEAVY WORKOUT #3

This workout should be done in 15 minutes, *excluding* warm-up.

1. Warm-up—60 jumping jacks.

2. Set a timer for 5 minutes. Do 10 Burpees, and rest for the remainder of the time on the clock. When the timer hits zero, reset for 5 minutes, and do 10 Burpees, and rest for the remainder of the time on the clock. If you do three sets, that's 15 minutes and 30 Burpees. You should be pretty wiped at the end—I was sweating and breathing hard after one set when I tested this just now!

If you need a reminder of how to do a Burpee: begin standing up, feet flat, arms at your sides. Raise your arms overhead and jump up, drop immediately into a squat, then put your hands on the floor in front of you, jump/walk your feet out behind you so you're in the pushup position, do a single pushup, jump/walk your feet forward underneath you, and leap up—one rep. If the text description leaves you confused, do a Google video search.

PRO TIP: Listen to your body and adjust all of this accordingly. This is *your* workout, *your* body, and *your* journey. I don't want you to hurt yourself, and I don't want you to feel like you're failing. *Any* movement at all is fantastic—heck, if you even just park your car a bit farther from the door and really truck it inside, that's winning in my book! Don't beat yourself up. One day at a time, stronger each day! On days I don't have a ton of time I often do interval sprints: 30 seconds on and 30 seconds off as fast as I can. This is great for fat burning and it doesn't take much time.

NOTE: Jack's advanced level workout is pretty darn advanced—I personally like to stick to the beginner or intermediate level. The great thing about these different levels is that if you have a workout buddy who's at a different level you can still workout together by doing some modifications or just doing fewer reps. Jack is in way better shape than I am, and he can lift heavier weights for longer, but that doesn't mean we can't still have fun working out together when we get the chance. Workouts go by much faster and are lots of fun when you have a buddy to laugh with. Strength training shouldn't be torture for you—try to enjoy it and challenge yourself. Do you have a friend, family member, or mate that really makes you laugh? That's the person you want in the gym with you. Don't be afraid to get silly and have some fun.

In closing, I would just like to wish everyone good luck with their #WilderWay2.0 journey, and add that I absolutely LOVE getting feedback from you as you progress. Send me before and after pics, send me measurement changes and weight loss numbers, send me your #WilderWay2.0 journey story. If you get stuck or have questions or just need support, the BGDIR Facebook group is a wonderful resource. There are FAQ posts, comment threads about all kinds of products, support and answers for international #WilderWay members, and more.

What follows from here are product and brand recommendations, tips and tricks, conversion charts, FAQs, a bunch of brand new recipes, and a workout music playlist.

Enjoy . . . and get your strong on!

BAKING AND COOKING SWEETENER CONVERSIONS AND TIPS:

Sweetener conversions:

Regular Sugar Stevia (blends)
5tsp →2tsp
¼ cup →1 TBSP + 1 tsp
1/3 cup → 2 TBSP
½ cup →3 TBSP + 1 tsp
1 cup →6 TBSP

I always sweeten to taste when I'm cooking and baking, and I'll even add a bit more so that it tastes sweet enough for me—I would rather it be too sweet than not sweet enough. If you're cooking for guests I would err on the side of sweet because most non-Wilder Way people tend to find our foods less sweet than what they're used to. When I recently made mini-cheesecakes for my daughter's 5th grade class, I made sure to add lots of sweetener. The kids were SHOCKED when I told them the birthday treats were totally sugar free.

Brown Sugar Hack: Just use your favorite favorite stevia blend. My current favorite is the Natural Mate with okra and pumpkin (no, it doesn't taste like either)—you can get it from Amazon—then add a teaspoon of blackstrap molasses. I use one cup of stevia to one teaspoon of molasses. This will work 1:1 with the brown sugar recipes.

This brown sugar hack was a life-saver for me when I modified our favorite Thanksgiving sweet potato recipe. I don't think you can taste a difference at all. If fact, several of my family members prefer my recipes with this modification! If this is too complicated for you, you can always order some Sukrin Gold from Amazon. You can also add some flavor extracts to kick things up a notch, but I usually don't.

For thickening, and replacing things like corn starch: Glucomannan and xanthan gum. I use approximately a 5:1 ratio of corn starch to xanthan gum. Xanthan gum and glucomannan can be used at a 1:1 ratio to start out and then go up from there as needed, depending on desired thickness.

PRO TIP: Not all sweeteners are created equally. I get so many messages about not liking a recipe and then once the sweetener is changed to one I recommend they can't believe the difference. My favorite sweeteners are *Natural Mate* infused with Okra and pumpkin. I find this one to have absolutely no aftertaste. You can find it on Amazon. I also like a mix of *Pyure* and *Swerve*. We love to add powdered *Swerve* to the top of baked goods. We also use a bit of Monk Fruit Extract, and we really like the Lakanto Maple Syrup as it really does have a similar consistency to regular syrup.

MORE OF JASINDA'S FAVORITE JAMS FOR #WILDERWAY WORKOUTS!

"City on Fire" by Tyler Batts

"Big Girls Cry" by Sia (Bleachers remix)

"Powerful" Remix by Major Lazer, Elle Goulding, and Tarrus Riley

"Birthday Cake" by Rihanna

"Shape of You" by Ed Sheeran

"Me Too" by Meghan Trainor

"Good Girls" by Elle King

"In the Name of Love" by Martin Garrix and Bebe Rexha

"Back 2 U" by Steve Aoki, Boehm, WALK THE MOON

"Say It" by Flume and Tove Lo

"You Look Good" by Lady Antebellum

"All Time Low" by Jon Bellion

"Drinkin' Too Much" by Sam Hunt (*hot nighttime workout jam) ;)

"Faded" by Alan Walker

"The Mack" by Nevada, Mark Morrison, Fetty Wap

"I Got You" by Bebe Rexha

"Cake" by Flo Rida, 99 Percent

"Castle on the Hill" by Ed Sheeran

"Solo Dance" by Martin Jensen

"Rockabye" (feat. Sean Paul & Anne Marie) by Clean Bandit

"Whole Heart" by Gryffin and Bipolar Sunshine

"Don't Look Down" by Martin Garrix (feat. Usher)

"Bounce" – Radio Edit by Calvin Harris and Kelis

"Run" by Tiggs Da Author and Lady Leshurr

"Alive" (Cahill Club Mix)—Sia

"Take Me Home" (feat. Bebe Rexha) by Cash Cash

"Move Your Body" (Single Mix)—Sia

"Sax" by Fleur East

"Love Never Felt so Good" (Fedde Le Grand Remix Radio Edit) by Michael Jackson, Fedde Le Grand and Robin M Christopher

JASINDA'S FAVORITE NEW #WILDERWAY FRIENDLY PRODUCTS!

Hydro Flasks ® and Swell Bottles ®—My family never leaves home without these. The kids have a set at school to use with their true lemon and lime.

90 Degree ® pants – I get these from Amazon. They are a great price and SO comfy. I've been known to wear them both in the gym and outside the gym under a dress. I love them!

Swim Suits For All ®—You just have to love a company whose motto is "Love every body. Beauty comes in all shapes and sizes, and so do our swimsuits."

Bowflex ® SelectTech Adjustable Dumbbells – These things are AWESOME! They are perfect if you prefer to work out at home. They only take a tiny bit of space and are all you need to begin lifting and challenging yourself by adding weights.

FLAVORGOD seasoning—Yes, these are pricy but we got a big set on a great sale and they really help make recipes versatile. Heck, how else can you easily make chicken taste 30 different ways? The bottles are large and last awhile. If you are going to try just one, start with the Ranch flavor.

Scout Bags—if you've done any of my life chats, you know that I carry an enormous tote bag filled with cosmetics, sweeteners, treats, nuts, Quest bars . . . whatever I can stuff into it. I just love these bags because they wear well and clean up easily. They have really fun prints and they come in every shape and size.

SPRI ® brand deluxe vinyl-coated kettlebells—these run from 5 pounds all the way up to 45 pounds, with each size in a different colored vinyl coating. They're great quality, not terribly expensive, don't take up any space, and can be used in a huge variety of exercises.

Extra Thick Yoga Mat—I've found that I really need lots of cushion when we are doing bodyweight exercises or yoga. Get a good thick one, or lay a few on top of each other so you're really comfortable. I love the Fit Spirit ® mat because it is extra thick and comes in cute designs.

Baleaf® Woman's Fitness Pocket running shorts—I wear as little as possible when I'm running and lifting because when I have my Sweet Sweat bands on it's just easiest. Sports bra, shorts, and the bands. These shorts are great!

BY REQUEST: JASINDA'S FOOD AND MOVEMENT DIARY

So MANY PEOPLE HAVE ASKED ME TO TELL THEM EXACTLY HOW much I eat and when. They want to know what I do in my workouts and when. What do I wear when I workout . . .

So below, by request, is an excerpt from my fitness and eating diary. Please remember a few things when looking at this:

I am six feet tall and I have a decently high muscle mass, so I eat a lot. You may or may not need similar amounts of food to keep your metabolism really moving. I've also found that, between my physical activity and my adrenal issues, I need to make sure I am getting in more carbs. That's just what makes my body feel good. You might find it's better for you to not eat as many carbs in your average day. Also, every body is different. Do what works for you and what feels good! Exercise and movement is secondary to your nutrition, so always focus on that first. Your foundation to good heath happens in the kitchen.

Breakfast:

I usually wake up between 5:00 AM and 6:00 AM. If I workout with Jack, we'll have something light to eat beforehand. Usually it will be toast, a few Wasa crackers, or nuts. We want to get our metabolism moving within an hour of waking up. If I workout out later in the day, I will usually eat my full breakfast and then workout mid-morning, after I get my social media and emails out of the way. A typical breakfast could include White Plate French toast with a side of yogurt and cottage cheese, or egg wraps. If we have a really busy morning, we might just have toast and a shake or yogurt. We try not to make things super complicated so we try to eat whatever we have in the house, and whatever is on sale that week and just make it work. If we find a great price on yogurt, we find ways to incorporate more yogurt into our meals for that week.

Workout:

When I work out with Jack we usually start with weights. I do more reps and sets of lighter weights, whereas Jack likes to do heavier weights and fewer reps. We love to do deadlifts, rows, swings, and presses. Then we try to do some metabolic conditioning. Jumping jacks, high knees, burpees, sprints, lunges, along with some dancing around and just being silly. Hey, sometimes we haven't had any coffee yet!

When I work out with Karri we usually do a nice outdoor jog, or we do some yoga mixed with some light weightlifting. If we want to get really crazy we sometimes do pull-ups or curls with the boy's empty Olympic bar. We do assisted pull-ups with resistance bands that make it much easier than the traditional pull-ups and curls the boys do. We also enjoy crunches or sit-ups—Karri and I like to push each other, as it's fun to have a workout partner to do these mini-challenges with.

When the kids are home on the weekends we like to include them in our physical challenges. My kids LOVE trying to do pull-ups or jumping jacks to fun music. We try to keep our workout time to 30–45 minutes max. You can spare that much time! It really is a small percentage of your day, and you are worth it!

Snacks:

We always have a post-workout snack. I like to do a shake, but if I am in a real rush I will just grab a protein bar, some yogurt, or a handful of lean meat.

Lunch:

Things are always busy in my house around lunch time. Jack and I are usually deep into work or meetings, so I always try to keep it simple. We usually eat soup, a sandwich or roll-up, or a nice big salad. I try to always have veggies or greens at lunch—we always have a tray of cut up veggies in the fridge so that on those really busy days we can just pull them out and munch on them. We generally have some meat for lunch, too. Being prepared and having things you like always ready in the house is really important. Don't put yourself in a situation where there are only bad choices; it might take an hour on a Sunday to prep ahead, but it will be worth it in the long run.

Afternoon snack:

My afternoon snack is always changing but it is usually something sweet. Sometimes I'll have a Dr. John's sucker, or a few caramels. Other times I might have a protein bar as I'm running to pick up the kids from school and take them to afternoon activities. In the summer I might have berries with a tiny squirt of fat free Reddi Whip. I ALWAYS keep lots of food choices in my purse so that if I'm on the go, and I really need a snack, I can just grab something and not be tempted by choices that wouldn't be as healthy or nourishing.

Afternoon movement:

If I've been on my butt all day I'll often take a break to do some squats, or a quick dance video. Sometimes I get on my walking tread-mill, or just do some quick jumping jacks. My job is pretty sedentary so if I don't take an afternoon break to at least stretch I can feel my body screaming by about 3:00 PM.

Dinner:

We believe it is really important for our family to be together at dinnertime. I'm so lucky that Karri helps me prepare meals most nights . . . so, so lucky. We always offer a salad, and a typical dinner for us would be bacon wrapped chicken, sweet potato sliders, a stir-fry or pasta and sauce. As I said in *BIG GIRLS DO IT RUNNING*, I think it is best to prepare the things your family already loves. Find a modified recipe—hello Pinterest!—or make some adjustments to what you usually make so that your kids and family feel happy and satisfied. Kids really need healthy carbs nightly, so I offer sprouted brown rice, pasta, or bread as a side.

Evening snack:

Yes, we almost always have something sweet at night. My favor-ites are some Dr. John's or Lily's chocolate, cottage cheese or yogurt with frozen berries and sweetener, peanut butter dip with a green apple, or a piece of dark chocolate. We might even add a nice glass of dry, red wine to our snack options depending on if it is a black or white day. If we don't get a chance to do our workout in during the day, we will often do that once we get kids in bed. In the summer months we love to do a run as the sun is setting, so if we do that we often have a protein shake as our evening snack. There is very little evidence to the fact that you shouldn't eat at night. I don't usually eat *right* before bed, but I see nothing wrong with an evening snack. If you're a mom like me, you deserve a treat just for getting through the day!

As you can see I EAT and drink A LOT! I don't deprive myself from good food or treats, and I'm the healthiest and strongest I've ever been. I don't think that you need to restrict calories or portions. You have a smart body! When you fill it with the right things it will let you know how much, and when, more fuels are needed.

BY REQUEST: JASINDA'S UPDATED GROCERY LIST

FOR YOUR PANTRY:
- Old-fashioned oats—I use these for so many things! Yes, steel cut oats are also okay.
- WASA crackers are so versatile! Use them with Laughing Cow cheese, veggies, berries, and even chocolate! I recommend the Rye and Sourdough flavors.
- Nuts, nut butters (no added sugar), and nut flours
- Brown rice—my family really likes the sprouted brown rice
- Quinoa
- Coconut oil. This oil is amazing! Pour it in your mouth, on your skin, and all over your food. Honestly, where has coconut oil been all my life? It's ahhhh-mazing!
- Extra virgin olive oil (for low and medium temperature cooking only)
- Spices—my favorites are ginger, cinnamon, cayenne pepper, pink sea salt (Pink sea salt is wonderful for you. We buy it in bulk on Amazon—amazing health benefits!), pepper, chili powder, oregano, garlic, turmeric, and basil
- Sugar- and chemical-free protein powder. We use Jay Robb.
- Mustard

- Apple cider vinegar—add this to your LaCroix sparkling water with some True Lemon. This is a tasty combo, sweet like soda but good for you; the health benefits of apple cinder vinegar are listed in the supplements section.
- Sugar-free pasta sauce; we *love* the Classico Riserva
- Dark chocolate (70% cocoa or higher), or stevia sweetened
- Pyure, Natural Mate, Swerve, monk fruit extract sweeteners, Sukrin Gold
- Seeds such as hemp, chia, and buckwheat
- Cocoa powder
- Coffee and tea
- LaCroix sparkling water
- True Lemon or True Lime

FOR YOUR FRIDGE:
- Power greens such as kale, Swiss chard, spinach, dark green lettuce. Salads are wonderful for lunch.
- Eggs—give us this day our daily eggs! These are the perfect food, so don't leave them out of your diet!
- Almond milk
- 1/3 fat cream cheese
- Oikos Triple Zero Greek yogurt
- Sour cream
- Cottage cheese
- All non-processed cheeses
- Mayonnaise (we are now eating the avocado mayo)
- Real butter—I recommend Kerry Gold
- Veggies
- Fresh salsa

- Lots of low-sugar fruits: lemons, limes, and berries are great for infusing into your water.

- Meat—I prefer to eat meat that is still on the bone. It has nutrients that boneless cuts do not have. Get some wings, thighs, or even whole chickens. My kids *love* wing night and we feel really wild and primal ripping that juicy meat off the bone.

FOR YOUR FREEZER:

- Meats of all kinds—it's really your choice. We stock up when things go on sale. Check your SAM's Club and Costco for good prices on organic meat. WE LOVE CHICKEN BACON! If you haven't tried that, I urge you to find some and give it a try. Super healthy and oh, so good!

- I *always* keep frozen berries to add to smoothies and our morning oatmeal mush.

- Frozen Spinach is great. Spinach is loaded with protein and iron and you won't even taste it in your smoothie—even Jack adds it to his post-workout smoothies, and he's told you how he feels about veggies.

- We also buy sprouted-grain bread and keep that in our freezer. Yes, these are expensive but I also buy in bulk when I see a good sale price.

- Frozen organic veggies (often cheaper than fresh, and just as good)

FRUIT AND SUGAR:

Yes, fruit has natural sugars, but some affect your body more than others. I'm not okay with cutting all fruit from your diet, because I believe God gave us these tasty treats for a reason. Just know that some fruits are going to be better for and easier on your body than others. Below is a list of the best and the worst fruits for keeping your insulin levels in a good place. And remember: all things in moderation.

- The best fruits: blueberries, raspberries, lemons, limes, avocados, and tomatoes. Two servings per day of these is fine.
- Okay-but-not-great fruits: green apples, kiwi, grapefruit, honeydew melon, mandarins, plums, peaches, pears, nectarines, strawberries and oranges. If you do choose these fruits try to limit them to one per day.
- On occasion fruits: grapes, cherries, red apples, pineapple, papaya, mangoes, and bananas. Because of the high fructose levels in these fruits they should be eaten very rarely.

BE CHOOSY WITH YOUR GRAINS:

Not all grains or carbohydrates have been created equally; some have a very negative impact on your body, and others are good for you. Most people are aware that things like regular factory-processed bread, cakes, cereals, cookies, and crackers are bad for you, but did you know barley and rye could have similar damaging affects on your body?

- The best grains: buckwheat, millet, oats, quinoa, brown rice, and flax
- Sprouted breads are always the best choice. You will find these in the freezer section of your grocery store.

JASINDA'S FAVORITE AND RECOMMENDED (UPDATED)

- Oikos Triple 0 yogurt
- Ezekiel bread
- Silver Hills bread
- Unique Sprouted Splits whole grain wheat pretzels
- Wasa crackers (Sourdough and Rye)
- Chunkie Dunkies cookies (the Stevia sweetened varieties)
- Applegate meat
- Lily's chocolate
- Dr. John's candies***
- Pur Gum***
- Jay Robb whey isolate protein powder
- Horizon Organics
- Laughing Cow cheese
- Crofter's Just Fruit spread
- Bragg's Liquid Aminos, ACV, and dressing
- Dreamfield's pasta
- Califia Farms milk and creamer
- Fairlife milk
- Bryer's Carb Smart ice cream and bars*
- Garden of Eatin' baked blue corn chips

- Hope Foods Guacamole
- Mary's Gone Crackers
- Mission whole wheat low carb wraps
- Joseph's low carb Lavash bread
- Kerry's Gold butter without canola oil
- Real Good pizza
- Kodiak power cakes – a great choice for the kids
- Quest protein bars*
- Kirkland Brand (Costco) generic Quest protein bars
- Bai drinks and soda
- Progresso light soup (non-cream based variety)
- Ezekiel cereal
- Wholesome or Plantation Blackstrap molassses
- Lakanto maple flavored syrup
- Primal Kitchen avocado mayo**
- Simple Girl sauces
- Uncle Sam's cereal
- PB & Me**
- FLAVORGOD seasonings
- Sir Kensington mustard and ketchup
- Organic Hope Guacamole
- Zevia soda
- Blue Sky ZERO soda
- Vitamin Water Zero
- Nut Pods creamer**
- Naturals Deli meat
- Sweet leaf flavored sweetener and water enhancer
- Naturally Nutty almond and peanut butter
- True Lemon and True lime water powers and flavors
- La Croix

- Natural Mate Sweetener **
- Pyure Sweetener
- Swerve Sweetener
- Bolthouse dressing
- Halo Top ice cream

*may contain sucralose

** we have only found these on Amazon

*** may contain xylitol, a sweetener that can be fatal to pets

PRO TIP: Go to the websites of your favorite products and sign up for their newsletters. For example, I often hear about how True Lemon, FLAVORGOD, or Lakanto are so much more expensive than similar items found in your local store, but if you can get a 40% or 50% off coupon (and often with free shipping) they aren't any more expensive at all. Sometimes I find they can be even cheaper and last longer than other brands!

WILDER FAMILY RECIPES...

#WilderWay Approved

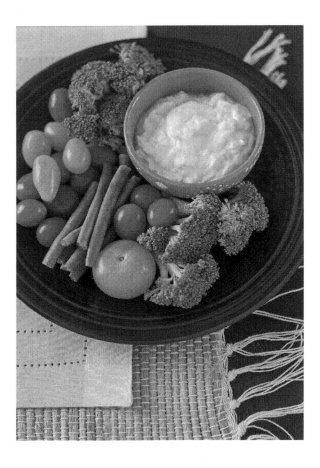

These recipes are some of our family favorites. Some have been modified from long-time family classics. Please note most of these will feed a family of 6–8 unless otherwise noted. If you have a smaller family, just halve the recipe, or save the remainder for leftovers—most things save really well in the fridge or freezer.

Wilder Way Pumpkin Cheesecake—Gray Plate

This a gray plate because if you're going to do a special treat you might as well go all the way. Right?

We usually use a pre-made whole-wheat crust, but you can also make an amazing pretzel crust using sprouted pretzels. Yum!

~Preheat your oven to 350 degrees

~Mix the cheesecake filling ingredients:

~3 (8-ounce) packages of 1/3 fat cream cheese

~3 large eggs

~½ of a 15oz can of pumpkin

~½ cup sweetener *I'll link the one we've been using below, but Swerve, Pyure, or a combo of both will all work. Always sweeten to your taste.

~2 tsp vanilla extract, or 1 tsp vanilla and 1 tsp pumpkin spice, (both will taste great)

~You can also add Lily's chocolate chips to the batter.

~Fill and bake for about 45 minutes to an hour. Keep an eye on it and cover the crust with tin foil if it looks like it might be getting too brown.

~Top with Fat Free Redi Whip, or drizzle melted chocolate on top after it has cooled. 'Cuz why not?!

It's just so decedent and so good! This is the perfect fall indulgence. Don't even feel guilty about it! #WilderWay

Strawberry Fried Cheesecake

Serves: 6

Ingredients:

~(1) 8oz package of 1/3 fat cream cheese, softened

~1/4 cup sour cream

~1 tbsp of your favorite sweetener

~1/4 cup sweetener (or to your taste)

~6 whole wheat Mission low carb wraps

~2 cups sliced strawberries

~1 Tbsp cinnamon

~1/2 tsp lemon juice

~coconut oil for frying

Directions:

In a bowl, beat together the cream cheese, sour cream, lemon juice, vanilla extract, and 1 Tbsp sweetener. Fold in 1 cup sliced strawberries. Divide the mixture between the 6 wraps. Fold up the wraps and use toothpick to secure closed. Brush coconut oil over the exterior of the wraps.

Combine remaining sugar and cinnamon. Roll wraps over in the cinnamon and sugar mixture.

Fry.

Remove toothpicks before eating. Serve with ice cream and top with remaining strawberries.

YUM!

Wilder Pumpkin Pancakes—white plate

Makes 40 large pancakes. Simply halve or quarter recipe to make a smaller batch. These will freeze well.

~4 cups of oats ground into oat flour (I do this with my blender first)

~2 containers of Oikos vanilla yogurt. Option: add or sub cottage cheese

~2 15oz cans of organic pumpkin

~4 cups egg whites

~4 tablespoons of sweetener—I've been using a new blend I'll link to down below, and remember: always sweeten to your taste!

~4 tsp vanilla extract. Optional: OR 4 tsp pumpkin extract

~8 tsp baking powder. Optional: additional 1 tsp pumpkin pie spice

~I always throw a few Lily's chocolate chips for the kids. They LOVE it as a very special treat.

Blend all ingredients in a blender and let sit for 10–15 minutes to thicken up.

Use coconut oil spray on your pan and cook on a very low heat.

Bacon, Egg, and Avocado Wrap – Black Plate

Hey, guess what? We actually eat avocado now! Who would have thought . . .

This is actually one of my very, very favorite black plate breakfasts now. There are so many good and delicious fats here that we use a bit of egg white and one of my most favorite chicken products . . . CHICKEN BACON! Yes, you read that right! If you haven't had chicken bacon before, you're missing out. Find it—find it now! Chicken bacon just might change your whole life. I will eat this for lunch or breakfast or any freaking time of the day because it is freaking delicious. If you don't love avocado just try this. Side note: my absolute favorite guacamole is made by a company called Hope. OMG, if you find that stuff, grab it and run. So, so, good!

Serves: 1

Ingredients:
2 Mission wraps
1 whole egg
1 egg white
2 slices chicken bacon, cooked
1 Tbsp cheese
¼ cup guacamole (optional)
handful of greens
1 tsp Dijon or spicy brown mustard

Directions:

Make some scrambled eggs with both one egg white and one full egg and then add your cheese. I love a nice sharp cheddar, but you can use what you like. Using a wrap, layer the mustard, guac, bacon and roll it up. You *must* try this! It is SO yummy.

Sausage variation!

Sub the chicken bacon with two links—or one patty—of cooked and sliced Applegate sausage.

BBQ Chicken Wrap

Serving: 1

Ingredients:
2 Mission wraps
2 oz cooked and chopped chicken
2 Tbsp Simple Girl BBQ sauce
1 cup lettuce

Dressing
- 1 Tbsp non-fat Greek yogurt
- ½ tsp FLAVORGOD ranch seasoning
- ¼ tsp lime juice
- pinch cilantro

Directions:

Mix together all dressing ingredients. Spread dressing on wraps and top with lettuce and chicken. Fold wraps and serve.

Cucumber Chicken Wrap

This is another one of my favorites! Something about mustard and cucumber is just magical.

When we are on the run I often make these wraps to go and just wrap them in foil. Don't get caught on the go without some yummy snacks in your purse. Yes, I would totally keep a chicken wrap in my purse—I'm a mom of six for goodness sake!

Serves: 1

Ingredients:
- 2 Mission wraps
- 2 oz cooked, cubed chicken
- ½ cup cucumber, chopped
- 1 cup spinach or greens
- 1 Tbsp plain Greek yogurt
- 1 Tbsp Dijon or spicy brown mustard

Directions:
Spread mustard and yogurt on wraps, top with chicken and veggies, roll up and enjoy!

Sweet Potato Sliders (Chicken)—White Plate

Serving: 1

Ingredients:
- 6 oz raw sweet potato, cut into rounds
- 1 slice cooked, turkey or chicken bacon
- 2 oz cooked, chopped chicken breast
- spinach leaves
- cream cheese chipotle spread
- 1 Tbsp cream cheese
- 2 Tbsp greek yogurt
- ½ tsp FLAVORGOD chipotle seasoning
- ¼ tsp FLAVORGOD ranch seasoning

Directions:
Preheat the oven to 400 degrees. Combine all the cream cheese spread ingredients in a bowl. Using a sheet pan, make the ingredients into sliders, using the sweet potatoes as the "buns." Bake the sliders for 20 minutes, and then flip and bake for 20 more minutes.

Sweet Potato Sliders (Beef)—White Plate

Serving: 1

Ingredients:
- 6 oz raw sweet potato, cut into rounds (I try to find the really big ones)
- 2 oz cooked, lean ground turkey or beef made into little patties
- 1 slice cooked turkey or chicken bacon
- spinach leaves
-thinly sliced tomato
- Cream Cheese mix:
Laughing Cow Cheese, flavor of your choice. I like the pepper jack!
- ¼ tsp FLAVORGOD ranch seasoning (optional). I often add this to the meat
- ¼ tsp FLAVORGOD ketchup seasoning (optional). I often add this to the meat

Directions:
Preheat the oven to 400 degrees. Combine all the cream cheese spread ingredients in a bowl. On a sheet pan, make the ingredients into sliders, using the sweet potatoes as the "buns." Bake the sliders for 20 minutes, and then flip and bake for 20 more minutes.

Simple and Spicy Soup

I think if you've read my first book you know that my family really likes things spicy. This soup is a family lunch favorite. I've been known to try and sneak in any and all sorts of veggies to see what I can get Jack to eat. I've even blended up some okra or cauliflower and snuck it in. Shh—don't tell Jack! If your kids like a particular veggie, start with those first. Bone broth is SO good for you! Making this once a week for lunch will help keep you healthy and strong.

Serves: 12

Ingredients:
- 2 lbs ground meat (lean and drained), browned
- 12 oz chopped veggies of your choice (we <3 celery and peppers)
- 6 tsp seasoning of your choice (we <3 FLAVORGOD garlic and cayenne)
- 2 tsp Himalayan pink salt
- 2–3 Tbsp hot sauce (Simple Girl is GREAT!)
- 10–16 oz Rotel tomatoes, or your favorite salsa
- 1 quart of bone broth
- 7 cups water

You can add a cup of cream and/or a few Tbsp of coconut oil to make it a black plate

Directions:

Brown the meat and then add the veggies and sauté. Add everything to a large pot (or crockpot) and let simmer for a while. You can garnish with cheese, sour cream, blue chips, Greek yogurt, and/or fresh cilantro.

The Amazing Frosty-Inspired Shake—White plate

Serves: 3

Ingredients:
- 3 cups almond milk
- 1 scoop vanilla protein powder
- 2 scoops chocolate protein powder
- 3 Tbsp rolled oats
- 1 frozen banana
- 2 Tbsp unsweetened coconut
- 3 Tbsp cocoa powder
- 3 Tbsp almond butter
- 1 ½ tsp vanilla extract
- stevia to taste
- 20 ice cubes

Directions:
Blend all ingredients well—without ice cubes. Once everything is well blended, add the ice cubes and blend until smooth.

Wilder Way PB Dream Bars—Black Plate

Oh my dear sweet baby goats, this recipe is *everything*. This recipe right here is worth the entire cost of this book. I could eat these things all day long and not even feel sorry. They might even need a subtitle like: If you are a woman on your period these might give you an orgasm! They are just that good!! I might even be eating one right now. ☺

Servings: Makes one 8x8 pan

Ingredients:
Crust—
- 1 cup almond flour
- 3 Tbsp sweetener of choice
- ½ tsp baking powder
- ¼ tsp salt
- 5 Tbsp butter, softened
- 1 tsp vanilla

Caramel Center—
- 6 Tbsp butter
- 6 Tbsp sweetener of choice
- 2 tsp blackstrap molasses
- ½ tsp salt
- 6 Tbsp heavy cream
- ½ tsp xanthum gum
- 1 tsp caramel extract

Fudge Topping—

- ¼ cup Lily's chocolate chips
- ¼ cup butter
- 2 Tbsp sweetener of choice
- 3 Tbsp heavy cream
- 1/8 tsp salt
- 1 tsp vanilla

Directions:

Crust—Preheat oven to 350 degrees. Place all ingredients in blender, pulse until well mixed and then pour mixture in an 8"x 8" pan greased with coconut oil. Bake crust for 15 minutes. While crust is still hot, spread 5 Tbsp peanut butter on top of crust. Cool the crust.

Caramel Center—In a sauce pan, combine all ingredients except heavy cream and xanthum gum. Once it's all melted, remove from heat, add cream and whisk. While whisking slowly, sprinkle xanthum gum over mixture. Mixture will thicken as it cools.

Fudge Topping—Combine all ingredients in sauce pan, whisking occasionally. Once all ingredients are melted and combined, remove from heat. Place mixture in fridge to cool; take out to whisk every couple minutes to make chocolate fluffy.

All together now—Once crust is slightly cooled, pour on the caramel sauce and place back in fridge. Once the caramel is slightly set, pour on the chocolate topping. Finally, put in the freezer or fridge to set.

Plain Old Cheesecake

Servings: Makes 2 pies

Ingredients:
- (5) 8oz packages low-fat cream cheese, softened
- 5 large eggs
- 1 cup sweetener (to taste)
- 3 ½ tsp vanilla extract
- 2 crusts of choice. I like to use store bought whole wheat crusts, but you can also make a pretzel crust.

Directions:
Pre-heat oven to 350.
Blend Cream cheese until smooth. Add in eggs, sweetener, and vanilla. Once it is well combined, divide evenly between the crusts. Bake for 45 minutes to an hour.

Option: Cherry pie filling is a great topping for this cheesecake! No need to bake it. Just mix the filling ingredients together and serve with the cheesecake

Cherry Pie

Servings: Makes 1 pie

Ingredients:
- 5 cups whole tart cherries
- 1 Tbsp xanthan gum
- ½ Tbsp gelatin
- 2 Tbsp blackstrap molasses
- 2 Tbsp sweetener of choice
-1 pie crust

Directions:
Pre-heat oven to 350.

In a large bowl combine cherries, xanthan gum, gelatin, molasses, and sweetener. Stir until well combined. Pour cherry mixture into the pie crust and bake for 1 hour and 20 minutes. Check on it periodically to make sure the crust doesn't burn. If it looks like it might, just cover crust with tin foil and finish baking.

Peanut Butter + Chocolate Protein Bites—Black Plate

These are another great grab and go snack. When you just need a little extra protein and something sweet grab a few of these balls out of the freezer and put them in your mouth.

Makes 16 bites (3 per serving)

Ingredients:
- 2 scoops chocolate protein powder
- 1 cup peanut flour
- ½ cup peanut butter
- ½ Tbsp FLAVORGOD chocolate donut
- 2 tsp vanilla extract
- 1 Tbsp sweetener of choice
- 2 tsp coconut oil
- 2 ½ Tbsp water

Directions:
In a large bowl, mix all ingredients thoroughly. I like to mix with my hands. It gets a little messy, but I personally feel it combines better that way. After it is combined, form the batter into 2 inch balls. Place your balls in an airtight container and place in the freezer.

Mini White Plate Snack

I've found it makes so much sense to keep things simple. I am taking a cue from the Europeans and the fancy restaurants and putting together a combo of yummy snacks on one plate. This actually closely resembles my kid's lunches some days. You can add some lean meat, wasa crackers or a wrap and you've got a meal! Veggies, protein, and dip! What more could you ask for?

Serves: 1

Ingredients:
- 1 green apple
- 3 oz deli turkey/chicken
- 1 cup carrots, sliced
- 1 cup snap peas, celery, cucumber, or peppers, sliced
- ¼ cup plain greek yogurt
- 1 tsp FLAVORGOD ranch

Directions:
Mix the yogurt and ranch seasoning to use as a dip for the veggies. Enjoy the deli meat and apple on the side.

Mini Black Plate Snack

Veggies, cheese, and nuts! What more could you ask for?

Serves: 1

Ingredients:
- 1 cheese stick
- 3 oz deli turkey/chicken
- 1 cup peppers, sliced
- 1 cup cucumber, sliced
- ¼ cup sour cream
- 1 tsp FLAVORGOD ranch
- ¼ cup nuts of your choice, unsalted is best

Directions:
Mix the sour cream and ranch seasoning as a dip for the veggies. Enjoy the deli meat, cheese stick, and nuts on the side.

Chocolate Cherry Capital Shake—White Plate

FUN FACT: Our closest major city is the cherry capital of the whole world! That means that if you are eating a tart cherry, it probably came from a tree pretty close to where we live. We have cherry trees on our property that we eat from all summer long. Yes, we spit the pits off the front porch, too. You can make this shake with sweet cherries too, but I am going to encourage you to support my local town and try and find the tart variety. It gives this shake a kick!

Serves: 3

Ingredients:
- 3 cups almond milk
- ½ cup oats
- 4 Tbsp cocoa powder
- 1 cup frozen tart cherries
- 4 scoops chocolate protein powder
- 2 Tbsp sweetener of choice
- 18–20 ice cubes

Directions:
Blend all ingredients minus the ice together, then add the ice and blend until smooth. Enjoy!

Sweet Potato Turkey Wrap—White Plate

I LOVE SWEET POTATOES!! They might even be my very favorite healthy carb. This dish tastes like Thanksgiving exploded in your mouth. I even have my picky husband eating it. He might make a face when he's doing it, but he eats it. Y'all know he loves it!

Serves: 1

Ingredients:
- 2 Mission wraps
- 2 oz sweet potato
- 1 Tbsp almond milk
-3 oz deli turkey
- 1 cup chopped spinach

Directions:
Cook sweet potato. Peel cooked potato and mash insides with almond milk. Lay wraps on baking sheet, spread sweet potato mixture on the wrap, and top with turkey and spinach. Broil for two minutes. Roll wrap up tightly and enjoy warm.

Tip: sprinkle a little FLAVORGOD ranch seasoning on the wrap before you roll it up. It's super yummy.

Chicken Bacon Salad—Black Plate

You can't go wrong with eggs and bacon. Ever.

Serves: 1

Ingredients:
- cheddar cheese
- 2 cups spinach, chopped
- 2 slices chicken bacon, cooked and chopped
- 1 hard boiled egg, sliced
- 2 oz cooked chicken, cubed
- Dressing –
- 2 Tbsp Mayo
- ½ Tbsp lemon juice
- ½ Tbsp Dijon mustard

Directions:
In a small bowl mix all dressing ingredients together. Set aside. In a large salad bowl or on a plate, layer spinach, chicken, egg, bacon, and cheese. Top with dressing and enjoy.

Italian Egg Scramble (or Omelet)

My two oldest sons wake up at 5:00 AM every school day because they leave to get on the bus before 6:00 AM. Often we come downstairs and smell the eggs cooking. Yes, these handsome boys can cook, too! All girls currently aged twelve and thirteen can send marriage applications to my attention in the year 2028. These next two omelets are 100% their experiment . . . I mean, recipe. This is what they came up with at 5:00 in the morning. Proceed with caution, but I did try it myself and thought it was pretty darn good!

Serves: 1

Ingredients:
- 3 or 4 eggs
- ¼ cup mozzarella cheese
- 1 Tbsp cream cheese
- 2 slices chicken deli meat
- 6 pepperoni slices, chopped
- hot sauce
- FLAVORGOD Italian Zest, to taste
- FLAVORGOD Everything Spicy, to taste
- FLAVORGOD Cheese flavor, to taste

Directions:

Scrambled Egg version: Whip the eggs and pour into a heated pan. Then just start adding all the other ingredients. Scramble altogether and enjoy.

Omelet version: Whip the eggs and seasonings together and pour into a heated pan. Once eggs are cooked on one side, flip, spread on the cream cheese, layer on the cheese, meat, and hot sauce. Fold in half and let the cheese melt. Enjoy!

Meat Lovers Egg Scramble (or Omelet)

Serves: 1

Ingredients:
- 3 or 4 eggs
- 1 Tbsp salsa
- cayenne to taste
- ¼ cup cheddar cheese
- 6 pepperoni slices, chopped
- 1 slice turkey, chopped
- 1 slice chicken, chopped
- 1 Tbsp cream cheese
- hot sauce
- FLAVORGOD Everything Spicy, to taste
- FLAVORGOD Bacon Lovers, to taste

Directions:
Scrambled Egg version—Whip the eggs and pour into a heated pan. Add in all the other ingredients and scramble altogether. Enjoy!

Omelet version—Whip eggs with FLAVORGOD seasonings and cayenne, then pour into a heated pan. Once eggs are cooked on one side flip them over and spread on the cream cheese. Place all other ingredients on top. Fold in half and let the cheese melt. Enjoy!

Jasinda's Fluffy White Plate Omelet

When I was in NYC with my oldest son we would go to a local farm-to-table restaurant each morning for breakfast. We ordered egg white omelets, and we were amazed with the giant, fluffy creation they would bring out to us. I've yet to get them as fluffy, but I can get pretty close. I toss my egg whites (usually 2–3 eggs worth each) into the blender with all of my favorite spices. My family is currently obsessed with FLAVORGOD ranch flavor. I blend it for about a minute and then pour it into the very lightly sprayed pan. (We want to keep this white so we need to keep the fats minimal.)

—Egg-whites
—salsa
—spinach
—laughing cow wedge (optional)

I put some yummy super food spinach inside with a bit of my favorite salsa. This breakfast is so filling, healthy, and nourishing. My husband always adds a bit of Laughing Cow cheese to his because he simply can't live without cheese.

Berry and Nut Salad

I love a nice salad for lunch, don't you? I usually just pile whatever I've got in the fridge onto the greens, but these are a few of our favorite combos. If you haven't tried the Braggs brand dressings, I would really urge you to try them. They are so healthy and light, perfect for this berry and nut salad.

Serves: 1

Ingredients:
- 2 cups lettuce/spinach
- ½ cup fresh berries
- nuts, few sprinkled on top
- blue cheese is optional especially if you are Mr. Wilder
- vinaigrette dressing
- 2 or 3 slices deli chicken or turkey, chopped

Directions:
In a salad bowl or on a plate, layer spinach, berries, blue cheese (optional), and turkey. Top with dressing and and a few nuts of your choice.

Easy French Toast—White Plate

When I released the first book a lot of people LOVED the recipe for the French toast sticks, and several people started eating them daily! I love that but sometimes I don't have the time to make them for the kids. Yes, they do freeze well but it seems like as soon as I make them, they disappear. If you have a French toast craving it's really easy to make a healthy version pretty quickly using sprouted bread. This is my go-to morning breakfast on my white days.

Use three pieces of sprouted bread. My favorite for this is the Silver Hills or Ezekiel cinnamon raisin if I want to feel really fancy.

Combine:
-1/3 cup Egg whites
- 1tbsp almond milk
-dash maple extract
-cinnamon and sweetener to taste

Mix well.

Soak the bread in the liquid. Place the soaked bread into a lightly sprayed pan on low heat. Be sure to flip and heat both sides.

Top with yogurt or cottage cheese and berries. YUM!

Taco Salad—Black Plate

Serves: 1

Ingredients:

- 2 cups lettuce/spinach
- 1 Tbsp guacamole
- 1 Tbsp cheese
- 1 Tbsp salsa
- 1 Tbsp sour cream
- ½ cup ground turkey, cooked and crumbled

Directions:

Place lettuce or spinach in a salad bowl, or on a plate. Top with turkey, cheese, guacamole, sour cream and salsa. Mix together and enjoy.

Cheesy Chimichanga

This one is a family favorite. My brother-in-law, a.k.a. The Marine, could eat 6 of these for dinner and still want more. If you like cheese, this one is a must-try.

Serves: 12 (yes, these freeze well)

Ingredients:
- 4.5 lbs ground meat (we use turkey or chicken)
- 24 Mission Carb Balance whole wheat wraps
- 4-6 onions, chopped
- bell peppers (optional)
- 3 teaspoons garlic salt
- 3 teaspoons taco seasoning (we use FLAVORGOD)
- 1 ½ teaspoons of pepper
- 3 jars of your favorite salsa (we like it HOT!)
- 6 cups of shredded sharp cheddar
- 6 cups of Monterey jack

Directions:

Cook the meat and onions and bell peppers, if using, and drain. Stir in all the seasonings and mix well.

Warm the tortillas and brush one side with olive or coconut. Spoon ¼ cup of meat in the center of an oiled side tortilla and top with 1 Tbsp of salsa, 1 Tbsp of cheddar, and 1 Tbsp of Monterey Jack cheese. Fold up the wraps and secure with toothpicks. Place in greased pan. Brush the tops of the wraps with oil and bake at 450 degrees for 10–15 minutes, or until starting to brown. Sprinkle with more cheese and bake another 2–3 minutes until the cheese is melted. Top with salsa, sour cream, and/or guacamole as desired.

White Plate Sandwiches

So many people worry about messing up white plates. I think it is best to try and keep it simple by just having one good serving of a healthy carb. Don't complicate things. Here are a few sandwich ideas that will maybe even inspire your inner sandwich artist.

Serves: 1

Option 1
Ingredients:
- sprouted bread
- deli turkey
- spinach
- FLAVORGOD seasoning of choice

Option 2
Ingredients:
- sprouted bread
- hummus
- spinach
- mustard
- tomato
Make a spread with the hummus and mustard. Top with spinach and tomato.

Option 3

Ingredients:

- sprouted bread

- 3 egg whites, cooked

- spinach

- Laughing Cow wedge

- FLAVORGOD Ranch

Mix laughing cow and ranch seasoning with egg whites. Top with spinach, or chop the spinach and mix with other ingredients—we eat this one open-faced.

Option 4

Ingredients:

- sprouted bread

- cream cheese

- cinnamon

- sweetener

- banana

In a small bowl combine cream cheese, sweetener, and cinnamon. Spread on one slice of bread, top with banana slices and add other slice of bread.

Wrap Inspirations

To make these extra special, grill them on both sides in a Panini pan, or in a frying pan.

Serves: 1

Wrap Option 1
Ingredients:
- Mission wrap
- deli turkey
- chicken bacon, cooked
- cheese
- spinach
- FLAVORGOD Ranch

Wrap Option 2
Ingredients:
- Mission wrap
- chicken, cooked and cubed or shredded
- spinach
- cucumber
- guacamole
- salt and pepper, to taste

Wrap Option 3
Ingredients:
- Mission wrap
- Laughing Cow wedge
- provolone

- guacamole
- spinach
- peppers
- deli turkey

Wrap Option 4
Ingredients:
- Mission wrap
- shredded cheese
- spinach
- salsa
- hot sauce
- chicken, cooked and cubed or shredded

Wrap Option 5
Ingredients:
- Mission wraps
- chicken, cooked and cubed or shredded
- guacamole
- mustard
- spinach

Wrap Option 6

Ingredients:

- Mission wrap

- chicken, cooked and cubed or shredded

- cheese

- guacamole

- cilantro

- salt and pepper, to taste

Wrap Option 7

Ingredients:

- Mission wrap

- 3 Tbsp plain greek yogurt

- ½ scoop vanilla protein powder

- 1 ½ Tbsp peanut flour

- 2 tsp sweetener

- ½ cup berries (fresh or frozen)

- dash of cinnamon

Mix yogurt, protein powder, peanut flour, sweetener, and cinnamon together. Use as a spread on the wrap. Top with berries. This one should not be heated.

Fancy Cheesy Wasa cracker

I made these crackers for a party and everyone literally RAVED about them. I know they might not sound very exciting, but they really are.

Serves: 1

Ingredients:
- 2 Wasa crackers
- cream cheese
- two thin slices of Leelanau raclette cheese
- Tuscan flavored olive oil (If you can find this, GET IT! Oh my word, it is too good to be true.)
- cherry tomatoes, cut in half
- salt and pepper, to taste

Directions:
Preheat oven to 350. Place Wasa cracker on a baking sheet. Spread cream cheese on Wasa, then add a slice of raclette cheese, brush with oil, and top with sliced tomato. Sprinkle lightly with salt and pepper. Place in oven for about 5 minutes. Enjoy this yummy treat warm.

Jasinda's Rise and Shine Shake

Blend together:

1 scoop Jay Robb Tropical Dreamsicle

1 scoop collagen

½ tsp vitamin C powder

½ tsp stevia

2 cups unsweetened vanilla almond milk

1 handful of frozen strawberries

½ of a container triple zero yogurt (I like banana)

splash of vanilla extract

Option: a handful of spinach or other greens

Jack's Chocolate Peanut Butter Dream Shake

Blend together:

Scoop of Jay Robb chocolate whey isolate protein powder

A cup or two of unsweetened Vanilla Almond milk (you can also use plain unsweetened almond milk and add vanilla extract)

Lily's chips, Lily's bar chocolate or other dark chocolate or cocoa—add as much as you want. I throw in about a handful of chips

One handful of frozen spinach

One handful of ice

One or two spoonfuls of natural peanut butter

You can also add additional stevia or swerve to taste

Ree's Fancy Strawberry Cupcakes

This was a special request for Nanny Karri's birthday, and then we used it for Baby Ree's 1ˢᵗ Birthday cake too! It was a big hit! You can top with fresh strawberries and make this a super duper fancy treat. (This could also be made into a cake.)

Serving: makes 18 cupcakes

Ingredients:
Combine and whisk dry ingredients:
½ cup almond flour and ½ cup coconut flour
1 cup oat fiber
1 scoop Jay Robb strawberry protein powder
2 ½ tsp. baking powder
2 T Puyre
2 T Swerve (always sweeten to your taste)
½ xantham gum
½ tsp salt
A few drops of natural red food coloring to make the batter a pretty pink

Beat wet ingredients together:
1 big spoonful of strawberry All Fruit
1 big spoonful of 1/3 fat cream cheese
½ cup salted butter, softened
4 eggs
1 cup water
¾ cup egg whites
½ tsp vanilla extract
1 tsp strawberry extract

Directions:

Add the wet ingredients to the dry ingredients and mix well.

Spread into muffin tins with liners.

Bake for 18–20 minutes

I let these refrigerate overnight and then frost them.

If these aren't sweet enough for you, you can always sprinkle more of the Swerve on top before frosting.

Frosting:

2 cups heavy whipping cream

1 generous Tbsp Swerve confectioner's sugar (always sweeten to your taste)

dash of salt

dash of vanilla extract

dash of strawberry extract

2 spoonfuls of Strawberry All Fruit Jelly

2–3 drops of food coloring to make it pink

Whip and whip it GOOD! This does take some time, but you want it to be a fluffy cream texture. I chill this frosting and then generously cover my cupcakes. You can add a bit of 1/3 fat cream cheese if you want the frosting a bit thicker.

Jasinda's Favorite Green Juice

I'm not sure if you've picked up on this yet, but I try to sneak in the good stuff—ie vegetables—whenever and however I can.

This juice is a favorite of our little Miss Ree Wilder. She will go to the cupboard and get out her special cup that we use just for this juice. Make some for your kids and see what happens. They just might become little green monsters, too!

Servings: 2–4
I like to use 2 bottles of cold BAI tea as my base.

Add one or two green apples
1 big spoonful of ginger
Juice of one lemon
Cilantro
A pinch of sweetener (optional depending on your level of sweetness)
1 scoop of collagen
Lots of yummy, fresh spinach and/or kale
Put everything in your blender and whiz away.
Option: If it is cold season I often add some powdered Vitamin C

Jasinda's Favorite Fancy Coffee

People are pretty serious about their coffee. In my Wilder Way challenge group, week 3 often brings about hysteria when people have to begin making changes to their favorite coffee drinks and, in particular, to their creamer. Most days I drink my coffee black with some collagen or MCT oil added—I'm just a beast like that.

If I'm at a fancy coffee place, I usually order an Americano. If have a sweet leaf caramel sweetener in my purse I might squirt a bit of that in, too. Jack was a Starbucks manager back in the day, and he is GREAT at making fancy, frothy drinks for me.

This recipe is just a simple hack I use to fancy up my coffee when I want to get really crazy. Sometimes you need a pick me up around 3 PM, right? And if you haven't yet entered the world of extracts, or sweetener drops, get on that now! They are magic!

> 1 cup of your favorite coffee
> 1 or two squirts of caramel extract, or you can use the sweet leaf drops
> 1 scoop of collagen
> MCT oil (optional and to your tolerance—I suggest building up slowly)
> 1–2 tablespoons of half and half, or cream
> additional sweetener to taste
> pinch of pink salt

I blend this all together, pour into a big cup and then sprinkle some cocoa powder or cinnamon or BOTH on top. You can also upgrade to real barista status by adding a squirt of Fat Free Reddi Whip. This is guaranteed to cure the sweet tooth, leave your skin, hair and nails fab, and keep your metabolism moving!

Jack's Favorite Tomato Soup

This is SO easy and SO tasty that is should be illegal.

Serves: 3–4

Ingredients:
- 1 jar marinara sauce (no sugar added)
- 1–1 ½ cups chicken broth
- ½ cup heavy cream

Directions:
Pour the marinara sauce and chicken broth into a sauce pan and bring to a boil. Once the soup boils, turn to a simmer and simmer for however much time you've got. Before you serve, add the cream and whisk.

White Plate Lemon Meatballs

These is another frequent request from my kids. I like to dip mine in marinara sauce.

Serves: Makes about 30 meatballs

Ingredients:
- 3 lbs ground turkey
- 3 cups brown rice, cooked
- 2 lemons, zested and juiced
- 2 Tbsp all purpose seasoning

Directions:
Preheat oven to 400 degrees.
Combine all ingredients in a bowl and mix.
Roll into balls and place on baking sheets. Bake in the oven for 45 mins, or until cooked through.

Bacon Mac and Cheese—Black Plate

This one doesn't even need an explanation.

Serves: Makes 1 8x10 pan, serves 8-10

Ingredients:
- 2 boxes Dreamfield pasta
- 8 Tbsp butter
- 2 cups half and half
- 2 eggs
- 1, 8 oz package of cream cheese
- 4 cups of your favorite cheese, shredded
- salt and pepper to taste
- cayenne pepper, garlic powder, and/or dry mustard to taste
- 2 lbs chicken bacon, cooked and chopped

Directions:
Preheat oven to 350 degrees.
Coat a casserole dish with coconut oil.
Cook the pasta as directed on the box, and then drain.
Add the cooked pasta to the wet ingredients, and then add the chopped bacon, and mix well. Pour the pasta mix into your casserole dish and place in the oven.
Bake for 20–25 minutes. It's done when it starts to bubble.

PB & J Oatmeal

My oldest daughter started making this, and then all of the other Wilder kids fell in line. They now ask for it every few days. If you need a comfort food, this is a great choice. If you want to keep it white vs. gray, just use some peanut flour instead of the butter.

Serves: 1

Ingredients:
- 1 ½ cup old fashioned oats
- unsweetened vanilla almond milk
- Oikos Triple Zero yogurt
- 2 Tbsp sugarfree peanut butter
- 1Tbsp no sugar added jam

Directions:
Place the oats in a bowl and pour over the almond milk until it just barely covers the oats (you don't want too much or it will taste watery). Microwave on high for 2 ½ to 3 minutes. Remove from the microwave, add in the yogurt, peanut butter and jam, and stir.

Pizza Wraps

BECAUSE IT'S PIZZA!! We like to eat it any way we can.

Serves: 1

Ingredients:
- 1 Mission wrap
- 2 Tbsp pizza or marinara sauce (no sugar added)
- ¼ cup mozzarella cheese
- handful of spinach
- 2 Tbsp chopped peppers
- 6 slices turkey pepperoni

Directions:
Spread sauce on wrap, top with cheese, veggies, and pepperoni.
Fold over all four sides and grill in a Panini pan, or in regular pan,
flipping halfway through.

Pizza Pasta

Serves: 8

Ingredients:
- 2 boxes Dreamfield pasta, cooked
- 1 jar marinara sauce (no sugar added)
- 2 cups mozzarella cheese, divided
- pepperoni
- 2 cups raw spinach

Directions:

Preheat oven to 350 degrees.

Grease 8x10 dish with coconut oil.

In bowl, combine cooked pasta, marinara sauce, 1 cup of cheese, and spinach. Stir mixture until well combined.

Pour mixture into a greased dish, top with cheese, and place pepperonis on top. Bake until cheese is bubbly and pepperonis are crispy, about 20-25 mins.

Pizza Chicken

Serves: 8

Ingredients:
- 2 ½ lbs chicken breast
- Italian zest FLAVORGOD (or your favorite Italian seasoning)
- 1 jar marinara sauce (no sugar added)
- 8 oz mozzarella cheese
- turkey pepperoni

Directions:
Preheat oven to 400.

Sprinkle chicken breast lightly with Italian zest.

Cook chicken on medium heat, on the stove, about 3 minutes each side. This just boosts their cooking.

Place partly cooked chicken in a greased 9"x13" pan. Pour marinara sauce on chicken, then sprinkle on the cheese and top with the pepperoni.

Bake for 20–25 minutes, or until bubbling.

Chicken Fajita Bowls

You can always find precooked chicken and rice in my fridge. I find that having those ready to go makes it so easy to whip together something quick. Chicken and rice can be boring, OR you can add a few things and you have a burrito in a bowl, or a stir-fry with a side of seasoned rice. A bit of food prep goes a long way toward making it easier for you to be successful.

Serves: 1

Ingredients:
- 1 ½ cups sprouted brown rice, cooked
- 2 oz chicken, cooked and cubed
- ½ a pepper, sliced and cooked
- ¼ sweet onion, sliced and cooked
- Toppings:
- a dollop of low-fat sour cream
- cheese
- salsa
- lettuce, chopped
- cilantro
- lime wedge

Directions:
Put cooked rice in a serving bowl and top with chicken, peppers, and whatever toppings you desire. Sprinkle your seasoning of choice on top, and squeeze on some lime juice, and you are good to go!

Jack's Lemon or Lime Pie hack

One night this summer I was REALLY craving some key lime pie. Sure, I could have gotten off my butt and made some, but you know how those cravings just hit you at 9 PM and you're too exhausted to get up and make a pie? No . . . just me? ☺ My husband came up with this excellent yogurt hack that is so easy you will be able to get up and make make it in just a few minutes.

Just take either a Triple Zero yogurt or Plain 0% Greek yogurt with a touch of sweetener and add some True Lemon or True Lime flavor packs. Yes, they do have packs that are JUST flavor without sweetener. You can find them on the website if you don't see them at your local store. www.truecitrus.com

Add some Ezekiel cereal and top with some Fat Free Reddi Whip and ENJOY!

Thank you, Jack!

Wilder Kids Candy Coated Popcorn

I splurge a bit at Halloween. My kids don't eat regular candy, so I make sure we have lots of Dr. John's Candies www.drjohns.com, and I always try to make them a special treat. Two years ago I got a special donut maker and found a few sugar free, low carb donut recipes on Pinterest and made those. This past year I wanted to try and do some fancy popcorn for them. We use a cheap air popper from Amazon that my kids love. Seriously, it makes the best popcorn!

Ingredients:

-Popcorn (we use non-GMO, organic)

-Seasoning of your choice: Ideas we've tried include cocoa (add sweetener), cinnamon sugar, FLAVORGOD chocolate, and gingerbread.

- ½ cup butter

- ½ cup blackstrap molasses

-1 tsp extract of your choice. We've used vanilla and caramel

½ tsp baking soda

Directions:

-Combine seasoning, butter, and molasses in a pot on the stove and heat to boil. Continue to stir for a few minutes.

-Take off heat and stir in baking soda and extract. Pour over popcorn and mix well.

-Lay popcorn on lightly sprayed cookie sheets and heat in the oven at 250° for about 20–30 minutes. Keep an eye on it and try to flip or stir once while cooking.

If you want to get really fancy, heat up some Lily's chocolate and pour that over the top, then let it cool. My kids RAVE over this treat. It tastes sinfully good.

Grilled PB & J

Hello, gray plate my old friend . . . My kids almost always eat gray plates because they now all have super healthy and speedy metabolisms. This is a favorite of the Wilder Kids. What kid doesn't love a good PB&J?

Serves: 1

Ingredients:
- 1 Mission wrap
- 2 Tbsp peanut butter (no sugar added)
- 1 Tbsp jelly

Directions:
Spread peanut butter and jelly on the wrap. Fold over all four sides of wrap. Grill on a Panini pan or in a regular pan, flipping halfway through.

Chicken Bacon Wrapped Chicken with Ranch

Serves: 6

Ingredients:
6 Chicken breasts
18 slices chicken bacon
4 oz cream cheese
4 wedges Laughing Cow Cheese
Ranch FLAVORGOD

Directions:
Preheat oven to 400.

In a small bowl combine cream cheese, Laughing Cow, and ranch seasoning. Set aside.

Place chicken breasts on a coconut oiled baking sheet. Make 3 or 4 slices in the chicken.

Spoon the cheese mixture into the slices in the chicken.

Sprinkle the chicken with more ranch seasoning.

Wrap each chicken breast in three slices of chicken bacon.

Bake in oven for 20 minutes, flip over, and bake another 15 minutes.

Turn oven to broil. Broil for 2–3 minutes on each side to make bacon crispy.

Holiday Sweet Potato Bake

Serves: 12

Ingredients:

    4 large sweet potatoes

    1 cup almond milk

    2 eggs

    1 cup sweetener of choice

    1 tsp salt

    1 tsp vanilla extract

    ½ cup sprouted wheat flour

    1 cup Sukrin gold (sugar-free brown sugar)

    6 Tbsp cold butter cut into pieces

    2 tsp molasses

    1 cup chopped pecans

Directions:

Preheat oven to 375.

Bake sweet potatoes for 35–40 minutes. Cut in half and allow to cool slightly.

Raise oven temperature to 400. Spray a baking dish with coconut oil and set aside.

Scoop the insides of the sweet potatoes into a large bowl. Mash the sweet potatoes, but not too much. You will want to leave a little bit of texture.

Now add the almond milk, sweetener, vanilla, salt, and eggs to the potatoes.

Mash together until well combined, but not smooth. You still want some of that texture.

Pour sweet potato mixture into oiled baking dish. Smooth out the top, set aside.

Directions for the Topping:

In a medium bowl, combine almond flour and Sukrin gold. Mix well. Using a pastry cutter, blend in the pieces of butter.

Add in molasses and pecans and mix until you have a nice crumble.

Sprinkle crumble on top of sweet potato mixture.

Bake in oven for 30 minutes, or until a nice golden brown.

Classic Pumpkin Pie

Serves: 1 pie

Ingredients:

2 cups pumpkin puree (1 15oz can)

2 eggs

1 Tbsp vanilla extract (if you want to get really fancy and spicy add 2 tsp vanilla and 1 tsp pumpkin spice extract)

1 tsp pumpkin pie spice

½ cup Sukrin Gold sweetener

1 Tbsp Natural Mate sweetener

1 Tbsp molasses

1 pie crust

1 Batch sugar-free condensed milk

- o 4 cups heavy cream
- o 4 Tbsp butter
- o 2/3 cup sweetener
- o

Place all condensed milk ingredients in sauce pan. Bring to a boil, reduce heat and simmer to reduce by half (about 30–40 minutes). Make sure to whisk occasionally to prevent burning. Should be thick and gooey when it's done.

Directions:

Preheat oven to 350.

In a large bowl combine pumpkin, eggs, vanilla, pumpkin pie spice, sweeteners, molasses, and condensed milk. Whisk or mix until completely smooth.

Pour mixture into a prepared pie crust, bake for an hour. Keep an eye on the crust. To prevent crust from burning place foil around edges if needed.

Cool completely and enjoy your yummy treat!

FAQS:

Q: Why does my weight stall when I start a new workout program? Or when I work out more?

A: Well, everyone is different. I've seen people totally stall when they increase exercise, and I've seen others maintain or shift weight to muscle, and yet others drop extra weight easily. The most common answer is that muscle takes up less room in your body, so often when we build muscle we also lose fat, but the number on the scale stays the same. As we start to gain more muscle we'll burn fat more quickly and we'll then see that number drop faster. But it does take time. Muscle isn't built overnight, and consistency is key. Keep measuring! Often we are losing inches even when we aren't losing weight. If the scale is driving you crazy, toss it or hide it.

Q: This is overwhelming and hard, there's no way I can do it.

A: That isn't really a question, but I hear this every single day. Yes, it is more difficult versus the mindless eating and lack of movement prevalent throughout most of America. But you *can* do it! Take it one day at a time, and one meal at a time. Try to simply modify the things that you enjoy to fit into the program. Do you like eggs for breakfast? Great! On white plate days, skip the yokes and add bread, on black days skip the bread and add some turkey or chicken sausage on the side. Don't make it harder than you have to. Take your time and do it right.

Q: Why is everything so expensive? I just don't think I can afford to live this way.

A: I know, I totally get it! I have a billion kids and they all *love* to eat. But, we've decided that just like a college education is an investment, so is healthy eating. We want everyone in our family to have a long and healthy life, and this only comes through making nutritional choices a priority. We cut back in other ways to make up for it. I would also add that our grocery bill has stayed the same, or even gone *down,* as the process has gone on. The costs of processed, pre-packaged, and fast food choices add up quickly, and you eat more of it because you're programmed to always want more. Real food is satisfying and doesn't run out as quickly. I also buy in bulk when things go on sale. I truly believe making healthier choices is doable at any income level, sometimes it just takes more planning and effort.

Q: I hate working out, running, lifting weights, and/or dancing. When will this be fun? Do I have to do physical movement with your plan?

A: I hate working out, too. You have to put on special clothing, you sweat, and then you have to take the special, now-sweaty clothing off. It's a mess. The good news is you'll feel totally badass and strong immediately after you finish. I usually go from hating working out to LOVING it about five seconds after we're done. I suggest trying to make it as fun as possible. Find a workout buddy, turn on your favorite music, get some workout clothes that make you feel good, and set rewards . . . anything you can do to make the time spent working out more enjoyable. We love to include our kids in our workouts when we can. It's inspiring to us to see them reach their goals and it pushes us to be better, too! If we make it a challenge, contest, or game, all of us have more fun. It doesn't get any easier, but it does become a way of life. I feel off when we haven't had our workout time, because it's now just part of our day. I'm praying you reach the same love/hate relationship with working out, running, or any way you get moving. too.

Q: What happens if I don't want to work out this week? Or if I'm on vacation, or sick?

A: Your nutrition counts for at least 80% of your overall health. Fitness really starts in the kitchen, so if you're struggling with sticking to both your workouts and healthy eating, I always suggest trying to focus on your food. You can also go back to the toning, sculpting, and "shredding" later. When you fall off nutritionally it will be much better to get both wheels moving again. You will feel much better sticking to your black and white days—or even individual white or black plates—and then jump back on the movement train when you're in the right place mentally. Just don't give up and totally throw in the towel. Make the best choices you can each day, at each meal.

Q: I really messed up and fell off the wagon, and now I feel like poop. What can I do to get back on track and feel better?

A: First, I suggest trying to do a mini-reset or detox. Several foods will aid in detoxification: cilantro, broccoli, kale, onions, garlic, lemon, water, cayenne, and apple cider vinegar will all help. If you've really overdone the sugar, a great way to curb the cravings you're probably experiencing is to make sure you eat lots of healthy fats, like avocado, nuts, and dark chocolate. These will help you feel satisfied and full. Make sure you get these in until you feel more stable, and on plan, and headed in the right direction with your choices. I believe those who succeed in life are often the ones who refuse to give up. New day, new choices!

Q: Is it okay to eat fermented foods?

A: Yes, I actually recommend eating some of those. Some of our favorites are traditional sourdough bread, pickles (insider tip: I might eat pickles nearly every day), vinegar, raw cheese, and yogurt! Jack says his favorite fermented food is beer. ((eye roll))

Q: Is it okay to eat and drink together? I've read conflicting information about that.

A: Well, to be honest, I've seen conflicting info on this, too. I do think you'll experience better digestion if you try not to drink at the same time as eating. Using your body's natural saliva and fluids to digest is best. I try to make sure to drink a glass of water before I eat and then drink again after. Sometimes that doesn't happen, or I just forget, but I do think you will feel better and digest better when you aren't chugging drinks during your meal. It will also help you know when you are full, and know the difference between hunger and thirst. I really feel more bloated when I drink my favorite carbonated drinks while eating my meal. If you have issues with gassiness or bloating, try to cut down on this habit.

Q: I pee when I run and or jump. What can I do about that?

*A: I am with you, Mama! I have the same problems. ☺ I often joke that jumping jacks are like riding the big slide at the waterpark—you never know which twist or turn might get you all wet. Seriously though, I do think that women who've had children should be able to run and jump. I found a great company called THINX that makes menstrual underwear and I use the sport version for workouts when I know I will be doing lots of jumping. These hold lots of fluid and I've never had an embarrassing issue when wearing a pair. I highly recommend them.

Q: What one thing is the most important? I am so overwhelmed by all you've told us.

A: I totally understand. This is a lot to take in, right? The most important first step is to detox from the sugar. I believe that is going to make the biggest difference with your health. If that takes you more than four or even eight weeks, that's okay! Just try and get as far away from sugar as you can. Focus on nutrition to start because that is absolutely the most important. Once you get a handle on that, then start moving. Start small and gradually increase movement and activity as you start to feel more confident with the #WilderWay plan. I whole-heartedly believe in the slow and steady approach. Take it day-by-day, and meal by meal. Even if it takes years to get there, you have a much better chance at having a healthy and happy life. It will be worth it.

Q: Do I have to drink wine?

A: No! You can drink whatever you like. I happen to like wine. A lot. But you can do a low-carb beer and most of the hard liquors, too. Just be careful what you mix it with. Bai or La Croix are favorites of my #WilderWay peeps who prefer mixed drinks. This is a plan that doesn't deprive you. There's no guilt on the #WilderWay! Relax and enjoy your favorite adult beverage. No judging here. I'll still be sipping my Cabernet Sauvignon like a classy lady until the day I die!

Q: Do I need to count calories or worry about portion control? What is the mathematical equation for success with black plates and white?

A: NO! Final answer. Please, for all things good and holy, stop that right now!! Spend your precious time counting your blessings, not points, carbs, portions, or calories. My best advice is this: Ingredients always trump portion nutritional values. Really take a look at the ingredients—does the product have added sugar? Fillers? Oils? Can you pronounce all of these things? Do the ingredients sound like they came from another planet? Don't eat it. We want the sugar to be naturally occurring. For white plates we want little to no fats. For black plate we want little to no carbs. Fiber helps to negate the impact of the carbs on your body. I look at all of these things when choosing foods that are good choices. I try to keep a nice running list of ideal choices in my Facebook group, and I've also listed our regular grocery list so you can look for these items in your local store. If they don't have it, ask if they can order it for you.

Q: How can I be successful when I'm out? What do you eat when you go out, or travel?

A: I talked about this a bit in the first book, but I think it's so important that it warrants repeating. I believe in creating a safety net in your health journey. Once you figure out what you really like and how to eat it in a way that promotes health inside and out, make sure that you don't leave home without a plan or a bag of treats. Get a nice cooler bag and make sure you have yogurt, meat sticks, cheese, nuts, a quest bar, chocolate, and/or a wrap if you are going to be out and you're worried about being tempted. When you go out to eat don't be scared to ask your server questions. Can you have sauce on the side? Does this have sugar added? Can I get this with a different side? What oil do you use? Can you use something else instead? My belief is that when you go out you are PAYING to have food prepared the way YOU want it. Don't settle for something that won't fuel your body, not to mention might make you feel yucky, too. Most servers and restaurants are very accommodating to allergy and dietary restrictions. Just ask! It's the #WilderWay!

Q: Will you have more plastic surgery done?

A: Maybe . . . maybe not. If I have anything else done it will probably be scar revisions from previous surgeries. I have two very large and gnarly scars that I would like to fix. One was from an infection and it caused a wide, dark, and sometimes painful hunk of scar tissue. The skin that bothers me the most is on my bottom half and, at this time, there honestly isn't a surgical procedure for removal of that skin that I'm comfortable with. Those surgeries can cause large scars and have a very high risk of infection. Yes, my body is already covered in scars, but I think at this point I've got enough. For now, I am very comfortable with my Spanx, Yummie Tummy, and compression pants to keep that skin in place. Jack is the only one who really sees that part of my body regularly and he's happy with things. Of course, I could always change my mind, but as of today, that's my feeling about my excess skin. I'll just tuck it and march on!

Q: I've been doing your plan for weeks and I haven't lost any weight. WTF?!

A: I hate when that happens. Here's what I've seen. This is very common in two types of women: those who have been dieting off and on their whole lives and have some very damaged metabolisms, and women who are dealing with menopause. I've found that in those two cases it can make months for the body to heal before it will start releasing excess weight and change its composition. My advice is to hang in there and trust me for a bit longer. It took some of my betas months before the scale and measurements started to really show the healing, but it *did* happen. Don't beat yourself up if it doesn't happen quickly. Give yourself and your body plenty of grace and time to heal.

Q: How can I figure out if a new product I've found in my local store is "safe" for me to eat?

A: It's tricky. Here's the easiest way I can explain it. First, with any prepackaged food, I am going to assume it isn't going to be a good choice because 80% or more of prepackaged foods aren't a good choice. I look at ingredients first. Does it have added sugar? Look for all 66 names, as sometimes they will list several. Then, I will look for chemicals, fillers, and oil. If it looks like it is clean from those then look at the carbs and fats listed. Remember that fiber negates the impact of the carbs and if you see carbs listed in a prepackaged item you will also need to see those fibers cancelling them out. We want little to no carbs for black plates, and very little to no fats for white. If all of that is still looking good, EUREKA, you may have found something! If you get stuck with this you can always email, PM, or post in my group. I am always happy to help investigate new products. My hope is that we will continue to see more, healthy, prepackaged foods. Until then, always err on the side of caution and try to stick to as many whole foods as you can. Remember that www.nutritiondata. self.com is my absolute favorite site for checking on the nutritional data of all whole foods. It's a great resource.

ADDITIONAL READING, RESOURCES AND COOKBOOKS:

The Food Babe Way by Vani Hari

Deep Nutrition by Catherine Shanahan M.D., with Luke Shanahan

Burn the Fat, Feed the Muscle by Tom Venuto

The Adrenal Thyroid Revolution by Aviva Romm, M.D.

You Are Your Own Gym by Mark Lauren

Anti Cancer by David Servan-Schreiber

100 days of Real Food by Lisa Leake

Crazy Sexy Juice by Kris Carr

Women's Running Magazine

Oxygen Magazine

www.authoritynutrition.com

SUGAR CONVERSIONS
FOR BAKING AND COOKING

Regular Sugar Stevia (blends)

5tsp $\longrightarrow$ 2tsp

¼ cup $\longrightarrow$ I TBSP + I tsp

1/3 cup $\longrightarrow$ 2 TBSP

½ cup $\longrightarrow$ 3 TBSP + I tsp

I cup $\longrightarrow$ 6 TBSP

"God meant for my body to be healthy and strong.
I am worth the time it will take to make myself stronger and healthier.

It won't be easy, *but it will be worth it.*
Yes, it's okay to do this for those who love me as well, but this is for me.
I was beautiful then, I am beautiful now, and I will be beautiful tomorrow.

I CAN DO THIS.

I can do this despite feeling like I can't, or that I've been told I can't.
My body is beautiful at any size.
My body is going to be unstoppable when I'm healthier and stronger, so watch out!
NOTHING WILL DEFINE ME.

Nothing will stop me.
I CAN DO THIS!"

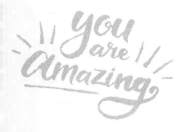

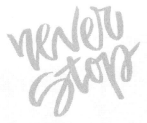

Grocery List

Oikos Triple 0 yogurt

Ezekiel bread

Silver Hills bread

Unique Sprouted Splits whole grain wheat pretzels

Wasa crackers (Sourdough and Rye)

Chunkie Dunkies cookies (the Stevia sweetened varieties)

Applegate meat

Lily's chocolate

Dr. John's candies***

Pur Gum***

Jay Robb whey isolate protein powder

Horizon Organics

Laughing Cow cheese

Crofter's Just Fruit spread

Bragg's Liquid Aminos, ACV, and dressing

Dreamfield's pasta

Califia Farms milk and creamer

Fairlife milk

Bryer's Carb Smart ice cream and bars*

Garden of Eatin' baked blue corn chips

Hope Foods Guacamole

Mary's Gone Crackers

Mission whole wheat low carb wraps

Joseph's low carb Lavash bread

Kerry's Gold butter without canola oil

Real Good pizza

Kodiak power cakes - a great choice for the kids

Quest protein bars*

Kirkland Brand (Costco) generic Quest protein bars

Bai drinks and soda

Progresso light soup (non-cream based variety)

Ezekiel cereal

Wholesome or Plantation Blackstrap molassses

Lakanto maple flavored syrup

Primal Kitchen avocado mayo**

Simple Girl sauces

Uncle Sam's cereal

PB & Me**

FLAVORGOD seasonings

Sir Kensington mustard and ketchup

Organic Hope Guacamole

Zevia soda

Blue Sky ZERO soda

Vitamin Water Zero

Nut Pods creamer**

Naturals Deli meat

Sweet leaf flavored sweetener and water enhancer

Naturally Nutty almond and peanut butter

True Lemon and True lime water powers and flavors

La Croix

Natural Mate Sweetener **

Pyure Sweetener

Swerve Sweetener

Bolthouse dressing

Halo Top ice cream

*may contain sucralose

** we have only found these on Amazon

*** may contain xylitol, a sweetener that can be fatal
to pets

Grocery List

Weekly Meal Planner

	breakfast	lunch	snack	dinner
SUNDAY	☐ white plate ☐ black plate	☐ white plate ☐ black plate	☐ white plate ☐ black plate	☐ white plate ☐ black plate
MONDAY	☐ white plate ☐ black plate	☐ white plate ☐ black plate	☐ white plate ☐ black plate	☐ white plate ☐ black plate
TUESDAY	☐ white plate ☐ black plate	☐ white plate ☐ black plate	☐ white plate ☐ black plate	☐ white plate ☐ black plate
WEDNESDAY	☐ white plate ☐ black plate	☐ white plate ☐ black plate	☐ white plate ☐ black plate	☐ white plate ☐ black plate
THURSDAY	☐ white plate ☐ black plate	☐ white plate ☐ black plate	☐ white plate ☐ black plate	☐ white plate ☐ black plate
FRIDAY	☐ white plate ☐ black plate	☐ white plate ☐ black plate	☐ white plate ☐ black plate	☐ white plate ☐ black plate
SATURDAY	☐ white plate ☐ black plate	☐ white plate ☐ black plate	☐ white plate ☐ black plate	☐ white plate ☐ black plate

The three possible plates for your meal

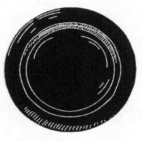

THE BLACK PLATE
Protein + Fat(s)

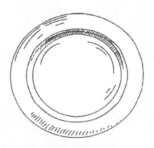

THE WHITE PLATE
Protein + Carbohydrates and starches

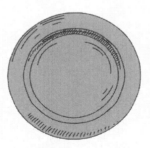

THE GRAY PLATE
Protein + Fat(s) + Carbohydrates/starches
(4-5 of these per week max)

FATS

nuts and nut butters
avocado
butter
cheese
cream
mayo
oils
whole eggs
full fat meats
chocolate
ice cream *
nut flour

*Bryers Carb Smart
and no sugar added coconut dream

Neutral Choices
UNLIMITED / EITHER PLATE

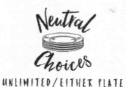

spices
lemons & limes
berries
asparagus
broccoli
cabbage
cauliflower
celery
cucumber
egg plant
green beans
all greens
mushrooms
onions
peppers
sprouts
squash
tomatoes (salsa)
zucchini
Dreamfields pasta
Okios 000 yogurt
Low carb/Whole wheat
Mission wraps

CARBS / STARCHES

sprouted breads
sprouted cereal
blue corn chips
old fashioned oats
apples
apricots
bananas
grapes
kiwi
melon
oranges/tangerines
peaches
nectarines
pears
pineapple
plums
popcorn
quinoa
rice (brown, wild)
beans
hummus
lentils
carrots
corn
potatoes (sweet)
WASA crackers (4)

Measurements

	arms	chest	waist	hips	thighs	lost
JAN						
FEB						
MAR						
APR						
MAY						
JUNE						
JULY						
AUG						
SEPT						
OCT						
NOV						
DEC						
total lost						

You are doing fantastic!

How I'm feeling

date:

place photo here

Hello
beautiful!

Exercise Log
Beginner

exercise	# of reps	total time	notes
jumping jacks			
pushups			
sit-ups			
1-minute plank			
30 sec side plank			
lunges			
squats			
straight leg lifts			
1-min wall sit			
high knees			
hip thrusts			
butterfly kicks			
mountain climbers			
jumping rope			

sprint distance: sprint time:

Workout Log

Mon ___   Tue ___   Wed ___   Thu ___   Fri ___   Sat ___   Sun ___

Exercises	Sets Reps Wt	Sets Reps Wt	Sets Reps Wt	Sets Reps Wt	Sets Reps Wt

I CAN DO THIS!

Journal

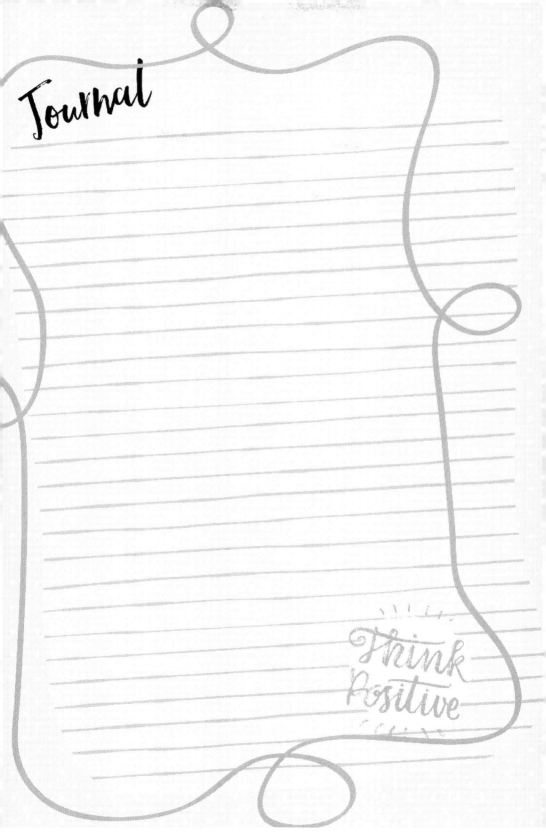

I WILL BE STRONG!

Positive mind,
strong body,
BEAUTIFUL LIFE

For printable versions of the worksheets: please visit,
www.biggirlsdoitrunning.com.

RECIPE INDEX